D0635580

CHURCHILL'S POCKETBOOK OF
Pre-hospital Care

*Dedicated to Tony and Henry, two very
personal patients, who continue to inspire
me in teaching others pre-hospital care.*

For Churchill Livingstone

Commissioning editor Timothy Horne
Project editor Jim Killgore
Design Erik Bigland
Project controller Frances Affleck
Page makeup Kate Walshaw

CHURCHILL'S POCKETBOOK OF

Pre-hospital Care

Matthew W Cooke

MB FRCS(Ed) FFAEM DipIMC RCS(Ed)

Senior Lecturer in Accident and Emergency Medicine
University of Birmingham and Walsgrave Hospitals
NHS Trust, Coventry

Member of BASICS-SoliCARE
(Solihull Immediate Care Scheme)

Member, Medical Advisory Committee,
West Midlands Ambulance Service

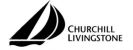

CHURCHILL
LIVINGSTONE

EDINBURGH LONDON NEW YORK PHILADELPHIA SYDNEY TORONTO 1999

CHURCHILL LIVINGSTONE
A Division of Harcourt Brace and Company Limited

© Churchill Livingstone, a division of Harcourt Brace
and Company Limited 1999

⟡ is a registered trade mark of Harcourt Brace and
Company Limited

The rights of Matthew W Cooke to be identified as author
of this work has been asserted by him in accordance
with the Copyright, Designs and Patents Act 1988

First Edition 1999

ISBN 0443-05987-X

British Library Cataloguing in Publication Data
A catalogue record for this book is available from
the British Library.

Library of Congress Cataloging in Publication Data
A catalog record for this book is available from
the Library of Congress.

Medical knowledge is constantly changing. As new
information becomes available, changes in treatment,
procedures, equipment and the use of drugs become
necessary. The author and the publishers have, as
far as it is possible, taken care to ensure that the
information given in this text is accurate and up to date.
However, readers are strongly advised to confirm that
the information, especially with regard to drug usage,
complies with current legislation and standards of practice.

Printed in China
EPC/01

CONTENTS

SECTION 3 TRAUMA

SECTION 4 MULTIPLE CASUALTY SITUATION

PREFACE

This book is intended for all those practising pre-hospital care. The first aider, ambulance technician, paramedic and doctor will all find the information applicable to them. Although every carer may not perform the skills and interventions described, everyone involved needs to be aware of them, so that we can work as a team. In pre-hospital care we are expected to be experts in every medical speciality's emergencies and give care in a difficult environment. If the individual cannot undertake a particular procedure, he should consider transporting the patient to someone who can or calling the person to the patient. What we must all remember is that the illness is not ours to treat, it belongs to the patient who simply wants it treated to the best of anyone's abilities.

This book balances the urgency of treatment with the limitations of the pre-hospital environment; an important issue rarely addressed in texts is the timing of transport to hospital. In each section, I have suggested when this should occur. In some circumstances this may not be possible, e.g. entrapment, or may not be appropriate, but these should be the exceptions which can be explained.

This book is designed for quick reference, either when treating the patient or when responding to an incident. The emphasis is therefore on treatment rather than diagnosis, which should be learnt before it is needed. It will also serve as a book to read in those inevitable long periods of boredom, whilst waiting for the next incident. The book is also designed to be used as revision notes for those undertaking examinations in pre-hospital care.

There is very little evidence for best care in the pre-hospital field. In some cases, evidence can be transposed from accident and emergency medicine; however the unique problems of pre-hospital care often mean that this is not appropriate. I hope that the information I have presented represents best practice. I would be interested to hear from anyone who believes that there is evidence to the contrary. It is vital that we all keep up to date. This book provides a basis of knowledge but it is your duty to keep up to date with the advances that often occur quickly in medicine.

ACKNOWLEDGEMENTS

I thank my many colleagues who have commented on the text and provided me with support in writing this book. I am grateful for all the assistance of the team at Churchill Livingstone and for all the help and encouragement.

Thanks also to the British Medical Journal and Resuscitation Council for permission to reproduce copyright material.

Most importantly, I thank Heather and Hannah for their support and patience during the preparation of this book. I hope they will see this book as a worthwhile result of all those hours spent playing on the computer.

NOTE REGARDING DRUGS

Whilst every effort has been made to ensure that all drug details and doses are correct, the author recommends that you should consult the British National Formulary whenever you use drugs with which you are not familiar.

Symbols used in the text

 Important points

 Additional notes

 Transport

Section 1

Principles of pre-hospital care

BEFORE YOU ARRIVE

Pre-call checklist
- Equipment (pp. 4–5) and drugs (pp. 154–169) should be checked regularly.
- Personal equipment ready ($\rightarrow$ p 3)?
- Vehicle ready?
- Replace everything at the end of each incident.
- Ensure fuel tank is always kept full.
- Recharge batteries on equipment.

Call checklist
- **E**xact location
  — find location on map before setting out
  — if responding alone, use familiar major roads rather than having to stop and check the map.
- **T**ype of incident.
- **H**azards, potential and known.
- **A**ccess to scene or rendezvous point.
- **N**umber of casualties/vehicles involved.
- **E**mergency services — response at present.

Note the use of ETHANE — the same system used in major incident reporting ($\rightarrow$ pp. 120–122).

- Put on protective clothing before starting journey.
- Think through possible actions whilst responding but not at the cost of concentrating on your driving!
- If you know children are involved, calculate size of equipment whilst responding (if you are being driven).

Attending the incident
- The standard of driving is the same for all drivers.
- You are responsible for your fitness to drive; think of new medication as well as alcohol.
- Never drive beyond your limits.
- Give clear, early signals.
- Plan your approach early.
- Change speed slowly.
- Watch out for cyclists, horses, etc.
- Always stop at pedestrian crossings.
- Be aware you are exempt from usual restrictions.
- You are still responsible for your actions.
- Make sure you are adequately trained.

Preparation Prevents Poor Pre-hospital Performance

DRESS FOR THE JOB

 Correct clothing is as much a piece of pre-hospital equipment as are drugs.

Checklist — clothing

- Green overalls.
- High visibility jacket with identifying labels.
- High visibility waistcoat with identifying labels.
- Identification tabard for major incidents.
- Boots with protective toe caps.
- Gloves — latex.
- Gloves — debris.
- Waterproof trousers.
- Fire resistant suit.
- Safety helmet with visor.
- Eye protection.
- Identity card.

Checklist — other personal equipment

This list includes equipment that each individual may wish to carry on his/her person, rather than in the equipment bag.

- Radio and spare batteries.
- Mobile telephone.
- Pager.
- Scissors/safety belt cutter.
- Torch.
- Report forms.
- Pens.
- Camera.
- Laerdal pocket mask.
- Stethoscope.

The day you forget to check your equipment is the day you are embarrassed at the incident.

MEDICAL EQUIPMENT

Airway
- Suction.
- Oropharyngeal airways.
- Nasopharyngeal airways.
- Bag-valve mask.
- Portable ventilator.
- Endotracheal tubes.
- Laryngoscope.
- Gum elastic bougie.
- Cricothyrotomy set.
- Tracheostomy tubes.
- Combitube.
- Laryngeal mask airway.
- Laerdal pocket mask.

Breathing
- Oxygen mask with reservoir bag.
- Oxygen supply.
- Long intravenous catheters for needle thoracocentesis.
- Chest drain.
- Flutter valve.
- Dressing with flutter valve.

Circulation
- Cannulae.
- IV dressings.
- Large bore (6 F) femoral cannula.
- Intraosseous needle.
- IV giving sets.
- IV fluids.
- Bottles for cross match.
- Fluid and line warmer.
- Splint for elbow.
- Field dressings.
- Syringes for drug administration.
- Needles.
- Skyhook for holding infusion bags.

Monitors/electronics
- Defibrillator.
- Sphygmomanometer.

- Non-invasive blood pressure (NIBP) monitor.
- Pulse oximeter.
- End tidal carbon dioxide monitor.
- Nebuliser.

Invasive procedures/dressings

- Scalpel.
- Sutures.
- Gauze.
- Antiseptic.
- Tapes.
- Bandages.
- Gel burns dressing.

Entrapment/immobilisation

- Femoral traction splint.
- Limb splints, vacuum or box.
- Semi-rigid collars.
- Extrication device.
- Spinal board.
- Vacuum mattress.
- Triangular bandages.

Patient protection

- Blanket.
- Waterproof sheet.
- Helmet.
- Eye protection.

Miscellaneous

- Triage labels.
- Forceps.
- Delivery equipment.
- Sharps disposal box.
- Cleaning tissues.
- Yellow clinical waste bags.
- Black rubbish bags.
- Water.

Now is the only time to restock, any later is too late.

SAFETY

HAZARDOUS CHEMICALS

 Safety always takes priority.

General principles of chemical incident management

- The Fire Service will take command.
- Stay clear of spilt chemicals.
- Keep other personnel clear.
- Medical priorities remain the same.
- If possible decontaminate at scene.
- If not possible to decontaminate at scene
  — wear protective clothing
  — isolate ambulance driver from rear of vehicle
  — open ambulance windows
  — wear BA in rear of vehicle if necessary
  — advise ambulance control and hospital of contamination risk.
- Arrange decontamination of ambulance.
- Dispose of contaminated clothing, equipment, etc. as advised by Fire Service.

Hazchem code. The Hazchem code (Table 1.1 and Fig. 1.1) allows rapid identification for the fire service on how to deal with chemicals. It can also assist in medical care. Full information is available from:

- Manufacturer, whose name and contact number will be on hazard information board.
- National Poisons Information Service 0121 554 3801.
- Fire Service.

BOMB INCIDENTS

Scene management
- Safety of yourself.
- Safety of the scene.
- Safety of casualties.
- Confirm the presence of a suspect device and its exact location.

Table 1.1
Hazchem code

1	Jet
2	Fog
3	Foam
4	Dry agent
P	Full protection, may be explosive. Dilute — safe to wash to drain
R	Full protection. Dilute — safe to wash to drain
S	BA required, may be explosive. Dilute — safe to wash to drain
T	BA required. Dilute — safe to wash to drain
W	Full protection, may be explosive. Contain, do not allow to enter drains
X	Full protection. Contain, do not allow to enter drains
Y	BA required, may be explosive. Contain, do not allow to enter drains
Z	BA required. Contain, do not allow to enter drains

- Clear the area
  — out of sight of the device as well as a safe distance
  — think of falling debris and secondary missiles
  — think of locations of secondary devices.
- Cordon off the danger area to prevent re-entry.
- Control the scene — this is the role of the police or military as soon as they arrive.

Special medical considerations

- Injury from blast wind causing disruption of tissues and amputation of limbs.
- Perforated ear drums indicate exposure to blast.
- Pneumothorax and blast lung.
- Think of injury from secondary missiles.
- Fragments in bomb cause other penetrating injuries.
- Crush injuries may result from masonry falls, etc. (→ pp. 111–112).
- Many may suffer psychological trauma; they should not be ignored because of the physically injured and counselling should be arranged.
- Remember to preserve forensic evidence and make careful records.

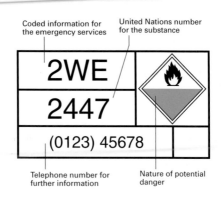

Coded information for the emergency services

United Nations number for the substance

2WE

2447

(0123) 45678

Telephone number for further information

Nature of potential danger

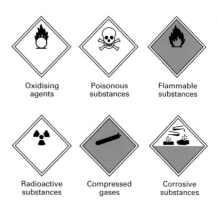

Oxidising agents

Poisonous substances

Flammable substances

Radioactive substances

Compressed gases

Corrosive substances

Fig. 1.1 Hazchem symbols.

Who needs to go to hospital?
- Injuries needing hospital care as in other incidents.
- Respiratory symptoms of any degree.
- Ear symptoms (bleeding, pain, deafness).
- Severe psychological distress after initial on scene counselling.

FIREARMS INCIDENTS

 The police are in charge at firearms incidents.

For known incident
- Check rendezvous point and approach by agreed route.
- Avoid lights and audible warning in vicinity of incident.
- Liaise with police officer in charge.
- Do not enter scene without specific permission.

For unexpected incident
- Drive away from scene if possible.
- If out of vehicle take cover behind:
  — substantial tree
  — thick earth bank
  — solid thick wall
  — engine block.
- Warn others who may be attending the incident.
- Keep everyone clear of the scene until the police arrive.
- Record details on paper or via radio as soon as possible.

Treating at the scene
Snatch rescue is all that should be undertaken in the danger zone. Even airway care and spinal immobilisation may have to be delayed if there is a high risk to casualty or rescuers.

What is a safe distance?
The largest distance you can achieve, including as much energy absorbing cover as possible.

Shotguns can kill at 150 metres, as can handguns.
No distance should be presumed to be safe.

- **A high velocity bullet can penetrate an ordinary brick wall.**
- **Beware of ricochet under a vehicle.**

Even if a bullet does not penetrate a ballistic protection jacket, the wearer may sustain significant blunt trauma.

Remember to preserve forensic evidence. Life saving treatment always takes priority over evidence but they are not mutually exclusive.

> *You are only of help to others if you are alive and fully functional.*

RAILWAYS

- Keep clear of the track unless vital.
- Contact signal box by railside telephone or via control; state
  — 'emergency call'
  — your name, ambulance service and callsign
  — exact location of incident
  — reason for power cut off.
- Train staff will be aware of safety equipment on train
  — circuit breaker
  — red flags/lights
  — warning charges.
- If possible request Railtrack to attend incident.
- Location can be given precisely using trackside marker peg numbers or gantry numbers.
- Current can jump one metre from live cable or track, more on a wet day.
- Always presume power lines are live.
- Always face the direction of oncoming trains or delegate duty to a spotter.
- Wear high visibility jacket.
- Place red marker or light on track if possible.

> *There is always another train coming.*

CIVIL DISTURBANCE

Unexpected

- Use silent approach and switch off emergency lights early when responding to any violent incident.
- Ask for police back up early.
- Always wear protective clothing.
- Ensure you are clearly identifiable and not dressed like police.
- When approaching casualty shout 'Ambulance Service' loudly and clearly.
- Remain calm, do not respond to aggressive actions.
- Watch everyone's hands (check both pulses as excuse for seeing casualty's hands).
- Wear stab proof jackets if provided.
- Work in pairs.
- Have one person stay in vehicle with radio if possible.

Expected

- Police are in charge.
- Find out rendezvous point and approach.
- Always wear protective clothing.
- Wear protective helmet with visor and eye protection.
- Ensure you are clearly identifiable and not dressed like police.
- Watch everyone's hands (check both pulses as excuse for seeing casualty's hands).
- Wear stab proof/ballistic protection jackets if provided.
- Only proceed forward under direction of senior police officer.
- Work in pairs.
- Have one person watch you as you proceed to call for assistance if required.
- If you are under threat, withdraw.

RADIO PROCEDURE

Numbers

1	wun	5	fiy ver	9	niner
2	too	6	six	0	zero
3	thuree	7	sev en		
4	fower	8	ate		

Letters

A	Alpha	J	Juliet	S	Sierra
B	Bravo	K	Kilo	T	Tango
C	Charlie	L	Lima	U	Uniform
D	Delta	M	Mike	V	Victor
E	Echo	N	November	W	Whisky
F	Foxtrot	O	Oscar	X	X-ray
G	Golf	P	Papa	Y	Yankee
H	Hotel	Q	Quebec	Z	Zulu
I	India	R	Romeo		

Accepted abbreviations

⚠ Only accepted abbreviations, understood by both sides of a conversation should be used. Remember, emergency services and hospital may use the same abbreviation for different subjects. Avoid medical abbreviations on the radio.

ETA	Estimated time of arrival
ETD	Estimated time of departure
RVP	Rendezvous point
Clear	Completed present case and available.

Short concise messages are all that are required.

INFORMING THE HOSPITAL

 Inform the hospital in any case where a team is required or critical time may be saved by avoiding delay after arrival.

If possible, direct speech contact with the receiving unit will decrease errors and allow clarification. A standard format:

- Ensures nothing is missed.
- Allows easy interpretation.

See also 'Calling the Trauma team' (→ pp. 116–117).

(→ pp. 116–117)

Content of message
- Age.
- Male/female.
- Type of incident and time of incident.
- Relevant history.
- Suspected diagnosis.
- Status of ABCDs.
- Active problems and treatment/interventions undertaken.
- Current status, e.g. cardiac rhythm or changes in ABCD status.
- Requirements at hospital.
- Estimated time of arrival.

 Call early with initial information and then update. At night a hospital may want to call staff in from home; this often takes 15 minutes.

All radio messages must be augmented by a concise verbal handover, which should be in the same format. Written records should be completed before leaving the hospital.

Early accurate information to the hospital leads to seamless care.

13

ON ARRIVAL

Parking at an RTA — other services in attendance
- Follow police instructions.
- Park near the casualty needing your attention.
- Do not obstruct ambulance access and egress.
- Do not obstruct fire tenders.
- Park between police cars marking the two ends of the incident.
- Park with wheels pointing to kerb, in case of a rear shunt.
- Doctor and incident officer usually park beyond the incident and the ambulances.
- Leave engine on and warning lights on.
- Particularly in urban areas, apply external steering lock or lock car doors with spare set of keys.
- Put on protective clothing.

Parking at an RTA — first on scene
- Park at a safe distance from the accident on same side of road as accident between approaching traffic and accident.
- Allow space for ambulances and fire engines:
  - Fire engines should be behind accident, unless safety or fire demands they are alongside.
  - Ambulances should be immediately beyond the accident.
  - Police will be at either end.
  - Allow space for them to enter.
- Park in fend off position.
- Leave all lights, hazards, beacons switched on.
- Particularly in urban areas, apply external steering lock or lock car doors with spare set of keys.
- Put on protective clothing.
- Go to far side of accident and make safe with cones, flashing light, other cars with hazard warning lights.
- Assess scene and report to ambulance control.

Motorway

- Principles are the same as for other accidents.
- High speed means greater danger.
- Allow greater distance between vehicles.
- Park beyond the incident.
- Never cross moving traffic on foot except under direct police supervision.
- If you need more room to work, get police to cone off an extra lane.
- When leaving scene, police will stop traffic before you pull out of coned off area.

Yellow jackets do not protect you if a car hits you. Make the scene safe as your first priority.

HELICOPTER

Role
- Remote incidents — poor access.
- Remote incidents — distant from definitive care.
- Allows bypassing of hospital lacking appropriate resources for the patient.
- Delivery of specialist personnel and equipment, allowing these to cover a greater area.
- Interhospital transfer.
- Maintenance of ambulance cover to an area whilst land ambulances are otherwise committed.

Disadvantages
- Noise — good communication between pilot, carers and patient must be possible within the aircraft. This can be achieved with appropriate systems.
- Vibration — although uncomfortable this is not usually of medical significance.
- Motion sickness — a major concern for the spinally immobilised or obtunded patient who is at risk of aspiration, particularly as head down tilt or lateral roll may be impossible.
- Anxiety.
- Space — smaller helicopters may not allow full access to the patient. Rear loading helicopters may not be able to transport the very obese.
- Flicker of blades may rarely induce fits in those prone.
- Cost.

Contraindications
- Late pregnancy, if left lateral position cannot be achieved.
- Psychiatric or behavioural problems.
- Recent fits.
- Decompression disease (although may be appropriate if flown at low altitude with no sudden ascent/descent).

Site preparation

The pilot will select the site most appropriate for landing. If you believe there is an obvious choice, contact the pilot and make the following preparations:

- Check that ground is firm.
- Clear area of loose debris.
- Keep people away and warn of dust in eyes.
- Ensure no animals in area.
- Switch off all strobe lights.
- Leave only sidelights on vehicles.
- Use flashing/rotating beacons only on instruction of pilot.

DO NOT

- Put up a windsock.
- Give hand signals to pilot.
- Illuminate area with headlights.
- Shine lights at helicopter.

Approaching the helicopter

- Do not approach the helicopter until signalled by pilot (a thumbs up).
- In general, do not approach until rotors are fully stopped.
- In emergency, crew will come to you.
- Always approach from the front.
- Never go near the tail rotors.
- Ensure that you have no loose clothing before approaching.

FIRE AND RESCUE

 The fire service is in overall charge of any area where there is a chemical, radiation or other major safety problem.

Services provided by fire and rescue service
- Control, extinguish and investigate fires.
- Fire prevention.
- Rescue/release of persons trapped.
- Rescue and control of chemical and radiation incidents.
- Make safe dangerous structures to enable rescue.
- Provision of special equipment at incident, e.g. lighting, boats, engineering tools, etc.

 If a piece of non-medical equipment is needed, ask the fire officer, who will often know a source.

Rank markings — epaulettes

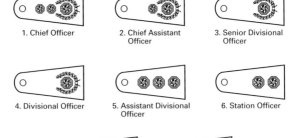

1. Chief Officer
2. Chief Assistant Officer
3. Senior Divisional Officer
4. Divisional Officer
5. Assistant Divisional Officer
6. Station Officer
7. Sub-Officer
8. Leading Fireman

Fig. 1.2 Fire service epaulette rank markings.

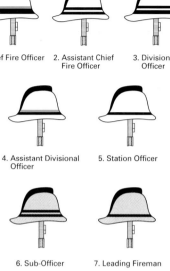

1. Chief Fire Officer

2. Assistant Chief Fire Officer

3. Divisional Officer

4. Assistant Divisional Officer

5. Station Officer

6. Sub-Officer

7. Leading Fireman

Fig. 1.3 Fire service helmet rank markings.

Liaison with the senior fire officer will make your job easier and decrease extrication time.

POLICE

Services provided by police service

- Control and coordination of all emergency services at scene.
- Control of public and traffic at scene.
- Safeguard property.
- Investigation of incidents, including collection of evidence.
- Escort duties.
- To act on behalf of HM Coroner.

Rank markings — epaulettes

1. Chief Constable

2. Assistant Chief Constable

3. Chief Superintendent

4. Superintendent

5. Chief Inspector

6. Inspector

Fig. 1.4 Police epaulette rank markings.

A senior police officer will often arrange transport of blood specimens to the hospital ahead of the patient.

DEATH

Pronouncement of death — criteria
- Decomposition.
- Decapitation or gross mutilation of body.
- Rigor mortis.
- Asystole present for 20 minutes despite resuscitation attempts.

Pronouncement of death — difficult areas
- Reported pulseless for 20 minutes or more.
- Ventricular fibrillation resistant to all appropriate treatment.
- Cardiac arrest in the elderly.
- Co-existing serious medical illness.

Cases where it is usually best to transport to hospital
- Cardiac arrest after penetrating trauma unless obvious devastating injuries.
- All children.
- Electrocution.
- Drug overdose.
- Hypothermia.
- Drowning.

In cases not listed above it is usually best to continue resuscitation and transport to hospital. There are occasions when it may be most helpful to discuss the situation with the patient's general practitioner who will have knowledge of the patient's pre-existing medical condition.

Living wills have no legal standing in the UK. It is important however, to recognise the ethical dilemma of continuing resuscitation in those in whom death is inevitable in the near future. It is important to involve the patient's relatives and doctor in such decisions. It is vital to be certain of the source of information on which you base such decisions.

Suspicious death
- The above guidelines still apply.
- Once life is pronounced extinct, there should be minimal disruption of the body and the scene.
- The police must be immediately informed.

- Any cannulae, endotracheal tubes should be left in situ, unless there is prior agreement of the coroner.
- No person is allowed to touch the body until the police are in attendance.
- The police will require examination by a forensic medical examiner.
- All procedures must be carefully documented.
- Your findings on arrival at the scene should be written down, as they may constitute important evidence.

The family

- Do not criticise lack of resuscitation.
- Do not falsely raise hopes.
- Prepare them for news of death.
- Do not tell them the patient has died until this is confirmed.
- Do not be impersonal.
- Families appreciate carers showing appropriate sadness and emotion.
- Offer advice on support available.

REFUSING EMERGENCY CARE

 **A significant number of those refusing
treatment have a serious diagnosis.**

Warning signs

If any of the criteria below are present, make a special effort
to convince the patient to go to hospital. If he/she still refuses,
ensure that the general practitioner is informed and that all
effort is made to explain to a responsible adult who can stay
with the patient.

Criteria:
- Disorientated.
- Decreased level of consciousness.
- Head injury.
- Pulse >110 or <40.
- Systolic BP <80 or >200.
- Respiratory rate >30 or <10.
- Inability to complete sentence because of difficulty
  breathing.
- Inability to walk safely.
- Chest pain or palpitations.
- Shortness of breath.
- History of drug ingestion.

 **Always stress that they should seek medical
help if their condition worsens.**

You may not need to transport:

- Diabetics who have recovered fully from a hypoglycaemia.
- Epileptics who have fully recovered from a fit.
- Persons with minor limb injuries.
- Third party caller emergency calls.

Section 2

Common medical problems

ANAPHYLAXIS — ADULT AND CHILD

Assessment

Skin. Diffuse itchy rash; urticaria; swelling, especially of eyelids, lips, hands and feet.

Respiratory. Upper airway: stridor; drooling due to difficulty swallowing. Larynx: stridor; hoarseness. Lower airway: wheeze; tightness in chest.

Cardiovascular. Tachycardia; hypotension; palpitations.

Causes:
- Foods, especially nuts.
- Insect bites.
- Chemical contact.
- Drugs.

Management
- *Remove the cause* if possible.
- *Adrenaline* 0.5 mg (0.5 ml of 1 in 1000) subcutaneously or intramuscularly if any respiratory or cardiovascular effects. (Although absorption is unreliable, it can be given without any delay.)
- *Clear the airway* and assess breathing.

 If airway is obstructed, consider needle cricothyrotomy. Intubation will only usually be possible by an expert with anaesthetic drugs.

- Give high concentration of *oxygen*.
- Give intravenous adrenaline 1 mg if cardiovascular collapse.

▪ If patient has respiratory or cardiovascular signs or symptoms, move to vehicle and continue therapy en route, unless transfer to vehicle will result in long delay. If airway deteriorates, specialist assistance will often be needed to intubate.

- ECG and pulse oximeter.
- Repeat *adrenaline* every ten minutes if required.
- *Chlorpheniramine* 5–10 mg intravenously.
- *Hydrocortisone* 200 mg intravenously.

- Fluid *volume* if patient becomes hypotensive. Give 500 ml colloid immediately and repeat as required.
- If there is marked bronchospasm, give 5 mg salbutamol nebulised with oxygen.

 If patient is on beta blockers and resistant to above treatment, give glucagon 10 mg IV.

CHILDREN

- Adrenaline 10 µg/kg (= 0.01 ml/kg of l in 1000).
- Hydrocortisone 4 mg/kg.
- Chlorpheniramine 0.2 mg/kg.

 Rapid administration of adrenaline is vital in anaphylaxis.

O₂

IM   Epinephrine   0.5ml   1:1000
                          (500 microgram

repeated in 5 min if no improvement

IM   10-20 mg Chlorpheniramine

if severe / recurrent / asthma
   100 - 500mg hydrocortisone
IV fluids   —   1-2 litres crystalloid

	7 11 yrs	6-11y	2-5yr	< 2y
Epi	500 µg	250 µg	125 µg	62.5 µg
Chlorphen	10-20 mg	5-10 y	2.5 -5 mg	
Hydrocortisone	100-500	100 mg	50 mg	

ASTHMA

ASSESSMENT

Features of life threatening asthma
Any of the following:

- Cyanosis.
- Exhaustion.
- Confusion, disorientation.
- Decreased conscious level.
- Bradycardia.
- Hypotension.
- Silent chest on auscultation.
- Unable to speak.
- Peak expiratory flow rate < 33% of usual best/predicted or unable to perform.

Features of acute severe asthma
- Cannot complete a sentence in one breath.
- Respiratory rate > 25/min.
- Pulse > 110 min.
- Peak flow < 50% of usual best/predicted.

Features suggesting a high risk asthmatic who may deteriorate rapidly
- Steroid dependence.
- History of previous sudden severe attacks.
- Previous ITU admissions.
- Multiple hospital admissions.

Features of mild asthma attack
- Can complete a whole sentence in one breath.
- Respiratory rate < 25/min.
- Pulse < 110/min.
- Peak flow > 50% of usual best/predicted.

TREATMENT

Life threatening asthma
- Ensure ABCDs.
- Administer 60% oxygen.
- Nebulised salbutamol 5 mg.

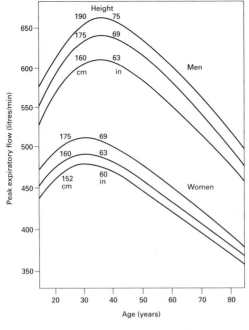

Fig. 2.1a Peak flow prediction chart (adults).

🗊 On scene time minimal. This patient may need treatment not available out of hospital, e.g. paralyse and ventilate. Inform hospital.

- Administer steroids
  — *either* prednisolone 40 mg orally
  — *or* hydrocortisone 200 mg IV.
- Monitor with ECG and pulse oximeter.

If not improving, use the following cascade:

- Recheck for another cause, e.g. tension pneumothorax, anaphylaxis.
- Continuous nebulised salbutamol.
- Intravenous salbutamol, 250 μg over 10 minutes.

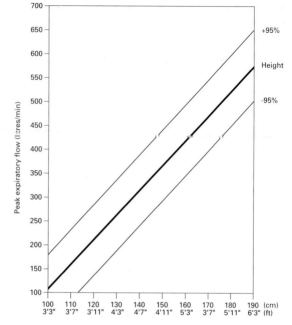

Fig. 2.1b   Peak flow prediction chart (children).

If in extremis:

- 1 mg adrenaline subcutaneously or intravenously will buy time.
- Intubate using ketamine anaesthesia.

 Anaesthesia in acute asthmatics is for experts only.

Acute severe asthma

- Ensure ABCDs.
- Administer 60% oxygen.
- Nebulised salbutamol 5 mg.
- Administer steroids
  — *either* prednisolone 40 mg orally
  — *or* hydrocortisone 200 mg IV.
- Monitor with ECG and pulse oximeter.

Recheck for another cause, e.g. tension pneumothorax, anaphylaxis.

If deteriorating:

- ▪ Transport whilst giving further nebuliser.
- Follow life threatening asthma treatment.

If not improving then use the following cascade:

- Give further nebulised salbutamol with 500 µg ipratropium bromide.
- Give prednisolone 40 mg orally.
- ▪ Transport and continue to monitor condition.

If condition improves after one nebuliser only, reassess condition:

- Condition still satisfies acute severe criteria — follow guidelines above.
- Condition satisfies mild asthma criteria
  — follow those guidelines
  — observe for 20 minutes
  — give 5-day course of prednisolone, 40 mg daily.

Mild asthma

- 2 puffs on inhaler if not attempted previously.

If not improving or unable to use properly:

- Salbutamol 5 mg by nebuliser.
- Reassess after 15 minutes minimum.

If worse or not improving:

- Give further nebuliser.
- Take to hospital or discuss with general practitioner.

If improved on one dose:

- Give advice.
- Ensure patient is left with responsible adult.

ADVICE BEFORE DISCHARGE

- Check patient understands medication.
- Check inhaler technique.
- Eliminate any new allergen source.
- Advise patient to speak to general practitioner or asthma nurse.

SEVERE CHILDHOOD ASTHMA

- First episode, consider foreign body aspiration.
- Think of anaphylaxis.

Assessment

Severe asthma if:

- Too breathless to feed.
- Unable to speak.
- Respiratory rate > 50
- Pulse > 140.
- Peak expiratory flow < 50% best/predicted.

Life threatening if:

- Peak expiratory flow < 33% best/predicted.
- Exhaustion.
- Decreased conscious level, listlessness.
- Silent chest.
- Cyanosis.

Management

- Allow child to adopt position of comfort.
- If treatment upsets child, this will worsen respiratory distress.
- Administer oxygen at highest concentration possible, if child is upset by mask ask parent to hold tubing near face.
- Salbutamol 2.5 mg nebulised via mask if possible.
- 🚑 Transport at this stage.
- Prednisolone 2 mg/kg orally
  — if unable to swallow, hydrocortisone IV.
- Aminophylline 5 mg/kg IV over 20 minutes, unless already taking an aminophylline preparation.
- Repeat nebulisers as often as required.
- If respiratory arrest
  — attempt bag valve mask ventilation
  — if this fails and intubation is impossible, try needle cricothyrotomy.

The commonest cause of asthma death is failure to recognise the severity of an attack.

BASIC LIFE SUPPORT — ADULT

Figure 2.2 below illustrates the Resuscitation Council's protocol for Adult Basic Life Support.

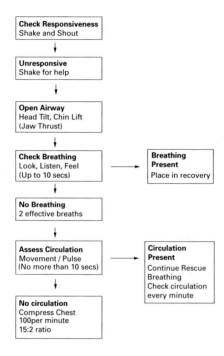

Fig. 2.2 Adult Basic Life Support.

RECOVERY POSITION

Below is the Resuscitation Council's protocol for recovery position in the unconscious patient.

> When circulation and breathing have been restored, it is important to maintain a good airway and ensure that the tongue does not cause obstruction. It is also important to minimise the risk of inhalation of gastric contents.
>
> For this reason the victim should be placed in the recovery position. This allows the tongue to fall forward, keeping the airway clear.
>
> - Remove the victim's spectacles.
> - Kneel beside the victim and make sure that both his legs are straight.
> - Open the airway by tilting the head and lifting the chin.
> - Place the arm nearest to you at right angles to his body, elbow bent with the hand palm uppermost.
> - Bring his far arm across the chest, and hold the back of the hand against the victim's nearest cheek.
> - With your other hand, grasp the far leg just above the knee and pull it up, keeping the foot on the ground.
> - Keeping his hand pressed against his cheek, pull on the leg to roll the victim towards you onto his side.
> - Adjust the upper leg so that both the hip and knee are bent at right angles.
> - Tilt the head back to make sure the airway remains open.
> - Adjust the hand under the cheek, if necessary, to keep the head tilted.
> - Check breathing.
>
> ### To turn a victim onto the back
> - Kneel by his side and place the arm nearest to you above his head.
> - Turn his head to face away from you.
> - Grasp his far shoulder with one hand and his hip with the other, at the same time clamping his wrist to his hip.
> - With a steady pull roll him over against your thighs.
> - Lower him gently to the ground on his back, supporting his head and shoulders as you do so; place his extended arm by his side.
>
> It is important to turn the victim over as quickly as possible whilst exercising great care, particularly not to injure his head.

ADVANCED LIFE SUPPORT

Figure 2.3 below illustrates the Resuscitation Council's protocols for Advanced Life Support.

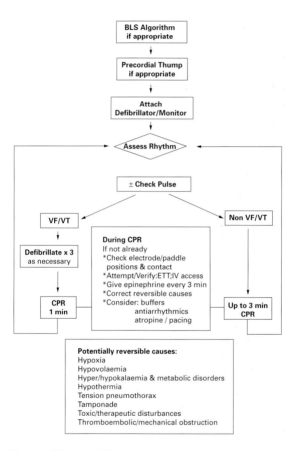

Fig. 2.3 Advanced Life Support.

BROAD COMPLEX TACHYCARDIA

Assessment/presentation
- Most patients are unstable with VT.
- Paroxysmal VT needs treatment.
- Difficult to differentiate from SVT with heart block.

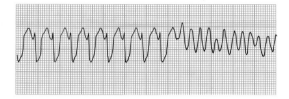

Fig. 2.4 Broad complex tachycardia.

Management if conscious
- Ensure ABCDs.
- If no pulse treat as VF, otherwise:
- Administer 60% oxygen.
- IV access.
- Adenosine if possible SVT with heart block ($\rightarrow$ p 37)
- Lignocaine 50 mg IV, repeated every 2–3 minutes up to 200 mg.

 Do not give lignocaine in torsade de points.

- 🚑 Transport to hospital.

Management if unconscious
- Ensure ABCDs.
- If no pulse treat as VF, otherwise:
- Administer 60% oxygen.
- Cardioversion 100 J, 200 J, 360 J.
- 🚑 Transport to hospital.

NARROW COMPLEX TACHYCARDIA

Pathophysiology

This must be of supraventricular origin.

Assessment/presentation

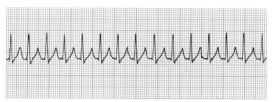

Fig. 2.5 Narrow complex tachycardia.

Management if stable

- Ensure ABCDs.
- Administer 60% oxygen.
- IV access.
- Vagal manoeuvres
  — Valsalva manoeuvre
  — splash ice cold water on forehead
  — unilateral carotid sinus massage
  — (avoid orbital pressure).
- Adenosine in stepwise fashion every 2 minutes if no response
  — start fast running IV 5% dextrose and give 50 ml bolus
  — 3 mg adenosine rapidly followed by at least 50 ml 5% dextrose bolus
  — 6 mg adenosine rapidly followed by at least 50 ml 5% dextrose bolus
  — 12 mg adenosine rapidly followed by at least 50 ml 5% dextrose bolus.
- ☐ Transport to hospital.
- Advise hospital may need urgent cardioversion.

Alternative treatments: (1) Verapamil 5 mg IV repeated twice if required (note, not to be used if patient is taking beta blockers). (2) Beta blocker.

> **Failure to correct may signify failure to recognise the cause.**

Management if unconscious

- Ensure ABCDs.
- If no pulse treat as VF, otherwise:
- Administer 60% oxygen.
- Cardioversion synchronised 50 J, 50 J, and 100 J.
- ☐ Transport to hospital.

BRADYCARDIA

> **Bradycardia can be the first presentation of acute myocardial infarction. It can also be evidence of fitness.**

Assessment/presentation

- Is patient stable?
  — check pulse, systolic BP > 90 mmHg
  — no evidence of heart failure
  — no chest pain
  — no dyspnoea.
- Previous episodes.
- Present medication, including beta blockers.

Causes include:

- Drug overdose — digoxin, beta blockers.
- Hypothyroidism.
- Hypothermia.
- Raised intracranial pressure.

If any of these are present then treat the cause not the effect.

Management
If stable:

- No new symptoms, refer to general practitioner.
- New symptoms:
  — give oxygen
  — 🔲 take to hospital.

If unstable:

- Ensure ABCDs.
- Administer 60% oxygen.
- Give atropine 0.5 mg IV.
- Repeat if no effect.
- 🔲 Transport to hospital.
- If no effect, give 2 mg atropine.
- If still bradycardic and unstable, consider external pacing.
- If patient is on beta blockers and unstable, consider giving glucagon 10 mg IV.

CHEST PAIN

> Chest pain can be the symptom of several life threatening conditions. An accurate history is often the most important factor in establishing the diagnosis. Presume a serious cause until actively excluded.

The type of pain is vital:
- Location and radiation.
- Nature.
- Exacerbating factors, e.g. moving, breathing.
- Precipitating factors.
- Associated symptoms.

The common serious causes:
- Angina/myocardial infarction.
- Pulmonary embolus.
- Pericarditis.
- Pleurisy.
- Pneumothorax.
- Aortic dissection.

> In pre-hospital care, it is not always possible to make a definitive diagnosis. In cases of doubt, treat for the most serious condition, without giving any treatment that would adversely affect your other differential diagnoses.

Immediate actions
- Check ABC.
- Give oxygen.
- ECG monitor.
- Pulse oximeter.

This section aims to help in the diagnosis.

Angina/myocardial infarction

> ↘ **Half the people who die of myocardial infarction do so in the first 2 hours.**

Cardiac pain
- Location — central or left sided chest pain with radiation to the left arm or jaw.
- Nature — tight crushing pain.
- Exacerbating factors — exercise. If pain occurs at rest, it should be treated as myocardial infarction until excluded.
- Sweating and nausea or vomiting are all highly suggestive of myocardial infarction.
- There may also be associated symptoms from the complications of myocardial infarction such as palpitations or heart failure.

12 lead ECG can be useful. In the early stages a normal ECG is of no significance. ECG changes of myocardial infarction:

- ST elevation.
- Q waves.
- Inverted T waves.

Location of infarct can be determined by location of these ECG changes:

- II, III, Vf = Inferior.
- V1, V2, V3 = Anterior.
- V4, V5, V6, I, aVl = Anterolateral.

Treatment: see 'myocardial infarction' ($\rightarrow$ p 63).

Pulmonary embolus
- Well localised chest pain.
- Knife-like.
- Shortness of breath.
- Haemoptysis.
- Collapse.
- Risk factors — immobility, local injury, contraceptive pill.
- Oxygen.
- Pulse oximeter.
- One dose heparin 5000 IU IV if certain of diagnosis.
- ⊞ Transport to hospital.

Pericarditis

- Angina-like pain.
- Worse with breathing.
- Worse on leaning forward.
- Pericardial rub.
- Non-steroidal anti-inflammatory analgesia.

Pleurisy/pneumonia

- Pleuritic chest pain.
- Cough.
- Shortness of breath.
- Fever.
- Analgesia.
- Oxygen.

Pneumothorax

- Sudden onset.
- Shortness of breath.
- Tall thin men.
- Hospital treatment after X-ray.

Aortic dissection

- Cardiac-type pain.
- Radiates to back.
- Worsening pain.
- Inequality of brachial pulses.
- Oxygen.
- ECG monitor.
- ◘ Transport urgently and inform hospital.
- IV line en route but no fluids unless profound hypotension.

Oesophageal pain

- Cardiac-type pain.
- Radiates to back.
- Worse on lying flat.
- Associated with waterbrash.
- Relieved by antacids.
- Treat at home only if certain of diagnosis.

Herpes zoster

- Pain in band corresponding to dermatome.
- Burning.
- Rash after few days.
- Oral acyclovir if certain of diagnosis.

Below is the Resuscitation Council's protocol for dealing with choking in adults.

If blockage of the airway is only partial, the victim will usually be able to dislodge the foreign body by coughing, but if obstruction is complete urgent intervention is required to prevent asphyxia.

Victim is conscious and breathing, despite evidence of obstruction:
- Encourage him to continue coughing but do nothing else.

Obstruction is complete or the victim shows signs of exhaustion or becomes cyanosed

If the victim is conscious:
- Carry out back blows:
  - Stand to the side and slightly behind him.
  - Support the chest with one hand and lean the victim well forwards.
  - Give up to 5 sharp blows between the scapulae with the heel of the other hand; each blow should be aimed at relieving the obstruction, so all 5 need not necessarily be given.
- If the back blows fail, carry out abdominal thrusts:
  - Stand behind the victim and put both your arms around the upper part of the abdomen.
  - Clench your fist and grasp it with your other hand.
  - Pull sharply inwards and upwards with the aim of producing sudden expulsion of air, together with the foreign body, from the airway.
  - Give up to 5 abdominal thrusts; if unsuccessful continue in cycles of 5 back blows to 5 abdominal thrusts.

If the victim is unconscious:
- Finger sweeps may be used to try to remove the foreign body.
- If this fails, give abdominal thrusts with the victim supine on the floor.

FOREIGN BODY OBSTRUCTION

There are a number of different foreign body obstruction sequences, each of which has its advocates.

If the child is breathing spontaneously his own efforts to clear the obstruction should be encouraged. Intervention is necessary only if these attempts are clearly ineffective and breathing is inadequate.

- Do not perform blind finger sweeps of the mouth or upper airway as these may further impact a foreign body or cause soft tissue damage.
- Use measures intended to create a sharp increase in pressure within the chest cavity, an artificial cough.

1. Perform up to FIVE back blows
- Hold the child in a prone position and try to position the head lower than the chest.
- Deliver up to five smart blows to the middle of the back between the shoulder blades.
- If this fails to dislodge the foreign body proceed to chest thrusts.

2. Perform up to FIVE chest thrusts
- Turn the child into a supine position
- Give up to five chest thrusts to the sternum:
  — The technique for chest thrusts is similar to that for chest compressions.
  — Chest thrusts should be sharper and more vigorous than compressions and carried out at a rate of about 20 per minute.

3. Check mouth
- After five back blows and five chest thrusts check the mouth.
- Carefully remove any visible foreign bodies.

Below is the Resuscitation Council's protocol for dealing with foreign body obstruction in children.

4. Open airway
- Reposition the airway by the head tilt and chin lift (jaw thrust) manoeuvre.
- Reassess breathing.

5A. If the child is breathing
- Turn the child on his side.
- Check for continued breathing.

5B. If the child is not breathing
- Attempt up to 5 rescue breaths, each of which makes the chest rise and fall. The child may be apnoeic or the airway partially cleared; in either case the rescuer may be able to achieve effective ventilation at this stage.
- If the airway is still obstructed repeat the sequence as follows:

For a child
- Repeat the cycle (1–5 above) but substitute 5 abdominal thrusts for 5 chest thrusts.
  — Abdominal thrusts are delivered as 5 sharp thrusts directed upwards towards the diaphragm.
  — Use the upright position if the child is conscious.
  — Unconscious children should be laid supine and the heel of one hand placed in the middle of the upper abdomen.
- Alternate chest thrusts and abdominal thrusts in subsequent cycles.
- Repeat the cycles until the airway is cleared or the child breathes spontaneously.

For an infant
- Abdominal thrusts are not recommended in infants because they may rupture.
- Perform cycles of 5 back blows and 5 chest thrusts only.
- Repeat the cycles until the airway is cleared or the infant breathes spontaneously.

DIABETIC EMERGENCIES

HYPOGLYCAEMIA

 Presume hypoglycaemia in any diabetic who is unconscious or behaving abnormally.

Pathophysiology
- Blood sugar < 2.5 mmol/l.
- Blood sugar is a poor predictor of symptoms.

Causes of hypoglycaemia:

- Excessive activity.
- Decreased food intake.
- Increased insulin.

Presentation
- Feeling hungry.
- Sweating.
- Vagueness, confusion, aggression.
- Fainting, decreased conscious level.
- Abnormal neurological status, e.g. hemiplegia.
- Hypoglycaemia causing events leading to injury, burns, etc.

Management
- Check ABCDs.
- Assess capillary blood sugar.
- If conscious and has normal gag reflex
  — oral glucose.
- If impaired level of consciousness or decreased gag reflex or rapidly decreasing conscious level
  — glucagon 1 mg IM or subcutaneously, unless prolonged starvation is cause
  — Hypostop (40% dextrose gel) into lower buccal mucosa with patient in recovery position
  — 25 ml 50% dextrose IV through free flowing IV line, then transport; repeat once en route if not improved.

Dextrose is more appropriate than glucagon if:

- **More than 45 minutes since onset of symptoms.**
- **Hypoglycaemia due to alcohol or drugs.**
- **Hypoglycaemia in non-insulin dependent diabetics.**
- **Glucagon already failed.**

☐ Transport is *not* required if all the following criteria are present:

- Full recovery.
- Capillary blood glucose > 5 mmol/l.
- Responsible adult who can care for patient for next 12 hours.
- Has taken some food since this hypoglycaemic episode.
- No other injuries.

If in doubt, treat the unconscious patient with IV glucose.

HYPERGLYCAEMIA

 Hyperglycaemia may be the first presentation of diabetes. Therefore the patient may not be known to be diabetic.

Assessment
- Vomiting.
- Polydipsia, polyuria.
- Illness in last few days.
- Gradual onset.
- Dehydrated.
- Drowsy.
- Raised respiratory rate.
- Smells of ketones.
- Missed insulin.

Management

- ABCDs.
- Assess dehydration.
- Administer 60% oxygen.
- Establish IV access and give 500 ml N/saline STAT if dehydrated.
- Transport to hospital.
- Maximum time on scene is 20 minutes.
- Reassess vital signs en route.
- Give further 1 litre N/saline over 15 minutes en route to hospital.

> **⚠ Avoid giving insulin before arrival in hospital, unless you have facility to measure serum potassium. Insulin can cause a catastrophic fall in serum potassium.**

In hyperglycaemia, the main abnormality to start correcting before arrival at hospital is dehydration.

The drowning victim is often protected by the primitive diving reflex. Complete recovery can occur after prolonged immersion.

Alcohol is often associated with drowning.

Management
- Your safety is paramount, do not take unnecessary risks.
- Ensure ABCDs.
- Clear airway.
- Remember that entry into the water is a high risk action for spinal injury.
- Start CPR if required.
- Administer highest concentration of oxygen achievable.
- Monitor ECG.
- Avoid giving atropine for bradycardia (the bradycardia is a physiological response and is protective).
- ▉ Rapid rewarming is best, therefore remove to warm ambulance and transport.
- Warm IV fluids if required, warm oxygen supply.
- Nasogastric tube as large quantities of fluid have often been ingested.
- Continue resuscitation until fully warmed, i.e. until after arrival in hospital, unless patient has obviously been immersed for many hours, e.g. bloating or putrefaction.

Early CPR and removal to a warm ambulance are essential in drowning.

DIVING ILLNESS

- Advice from Fort Bovisand, Plymouth 01752 261910.
- Decompression illness related to depth, duration and activity during dive, speed of ascent.
- Presentations of decompression
  — joint pain = the bends
  — skin = the itches
  — pulmonary
  — neurological.
- Barotrauma to lungs causing pneumothorax, emphysema, arterial gas embolism.
- Treatment
  — 100% oxygen
  — recompression as rapidly as possible.
- Helicopter transfer is acceptable if altitude is kept low and sudden changes in altitude are avoided.

ECG INTERPRETATION

 Treat the patient, not the ECG.

 Look for a treatable cause of the abnormality:
- Hypoxia.
- Acidosis.
- Hypotension/hypovolaemia.

Simply follow this algorithm to allow easy ECG rhythm recognition.

1. Is there any electrical activity?
   - If yes, go to 2
   - If no, check leads and gain, if no change → ASYSTOLE

2. Are there any recognisable patterns or complexes?
   - If yes, go to 3
   - If no → VENTRICULAR FIBRILLATION

3. Is a pulse palpable?
   - If yes, go to 4
   - If no
       3.1 Is it a broad complex and fast?
           - If yes → VENTRICULAR TACHYCARDIA
           - If no → PULSELESS ELECTRICAL ACTIVITY (aka ELECTROMECHANICAL DISSOCIATION)

4. How fast is the heart rate?
   - If > 100 tachycardia
   - If < 60 bradycardia

5. Are there P waves present?
   - If no
       5.1 Are there broad complexes with a tachycardia?
           → VENTRICULAR TACHYCARDIA
       5.2 Is it irregular? → ATRIAL FIBRILLATION
       5.3 Are complexes normal appearance and regular?
           → JUNCTIONAL RHYTHM

6. Is P wave rate approximately 300?
   - If yes → ATRIAL FLUTTER
   - If no, proceed to 7

7. Is there only one P wave for each QRS?
   - If yes
     7.1 Is pulse less than 150?
       - If yes → SINUS RHYTHM
       - If no → SUPRAVENTRICULAR
         TACHYCARDIA
       - If no, then proceed to 8

8. Are there the same number of P waves as QRS?
   - If yes, and PR interval > 5 small squares
     → 1st Degree heart block
   - If no, proceed to 9

9. Is PR rate constant?
   - If yes and RR variable → 2nd Degree type II heart block
   - If no, go to 10

10. Is RR variable?
    - If yes → 2nd Degree type I heart block
    - If no, and P and QRS completely dissociated
      → 3rd Degree heart block

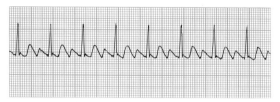

Atrial flutter

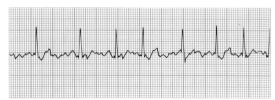

Atrial fibrillation

Fig. 2.6 Common ECG patterns.

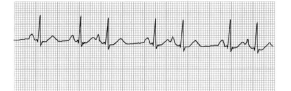

Atrial ectopics

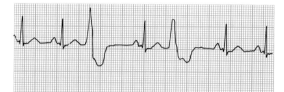

Ventricular ectopics

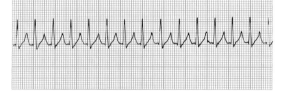

Supraventricular tachycardia

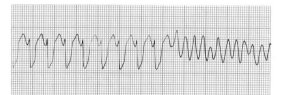

Ventricular tachycardia and fibrillation

Fig. 2.6 *(cont'd)*   Common ECG patterns.

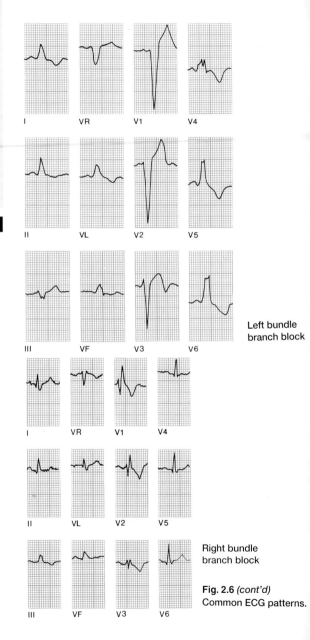

Left bundle branch block

Right bundle branch block

Fig. 2.6 *(cont'd)* Common ECG patterns.

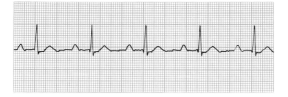

First degree heart block

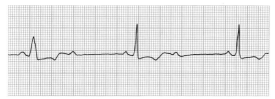

Second degree heart block (Mobitz type I or Wenckebach)

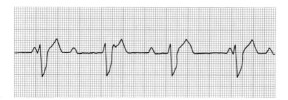

Second degree heart block (Mobitz type II)

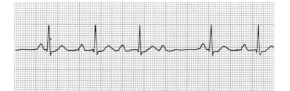

Complete (third degree) heart block

Fig. 2.6 *(cont'd)* Common ECG patterns.

ELECTROCUTION

Pathophysiology
- Domestic voltage may produce early arrhythmias.
- Higher voltage may produce arrhythmias in first 24–48 hours.
- Sustained muscle spasm may prevent breathing.
- Skin burns may be the tip of the iceberg — damage to muscles and nerves may be life threatening.

Management
- Safety — ensure power supply is off and will remain off.

> **Electricity supply companies will routinely reconnect supply after 20 minutes unless informed.**

- Follow ABCs.
- Connect to ECG monitor as soon as possible.
- ☐ Transport to hospital early in view of risk of cardiac dysrhythmias.
- ☐ Take to nearest A&E, not burns unit, in view of myocardial problems.
- Small surface burns may hide extensive deep tissue burning.
- Give 1 litre Hartmann's STAT if high voltage burn or muscle tenderness proximal to burn (to produce diuresis and decrease effects of myoglobinuria).
- Circumferential burns may compromise circulation.
- Observe for evidence of imparied circulation due to compartment syndrome.
- Effects of burnt muscle may be similar to crush syndrome (→ p 111):
  — hyperkalaemia
  — acidosis
  — myoglobinaemia
  — hypocalcaemia.
- Elevate affected limbs.
- Apply cling film to burns.

FITS

 Always look for a cause of the fit. Never presume it is epilepsy.

Causes
- Fever in children.
- Cerebral hypoxia, e.g. cardiac arrest, respiratory problems.
- Cerebral perfusion deficit, e.g. systemic hypotension, arrhythmia.
- Head injury (→ pp. 100–102).
- Hypoglycaemia (→ p 46).
- Meningitis (→ p 62).
- Drugs.
- Eclampsia (→ p 74).

Management
- Protect patient from further injury.
- Ensure ABCDs.
- If airway remains obstructed, gently insert well lubricated naso-pharyngeal airway.
- Administer 60% oxygen.

If fitting persists for more than 5 minutes:

- Obtain IV access.
- Check capillary blood sugar.
- Diazemuls 5–10 mg IV slowly (or 10 mg rectal).
- Repeat if still fitting after 3–5 minutes.

If fitting continues consider:

- Paraldehyde (0.3 ml/kg rectally) diluted in saline.
- ◼ If possible to evacuate, then do so at this stage.
- Phenytoin 15 mg/kg over 20 minutes (unless already taking phenytoin).
- Thiopentone anaesthesia.

◼ When carrying a fitting or postictal patient to the ambulance:

- Have patient on oxygen.
- Have good suction available.
- Monitor pulse and respiration.
- Use pulse oximeter if possible.
- Use a scoop or spinal board rather than a chair, in case adverse event occurs.

FEBRILE CONVULSION

 Always look for a cause of the fit.
Always consider meningitis.

Diagnosis
- Usually age 3 months to 5 years.
- Often unwell before fit.
- Generalised non-focal fit.
- No residual weakness.

If abnormal features, consider other diagnosis:

- Look for non-blanching rash or meningism.
- Look for signs of injury.
- Consider poisoning.
- Consider hypoglycaemia.

Management
- Undress the child.
- Tepid sponge.
- If fit not stopped in 3–4 minutes, give rectal diazepam:
  — under one year of age 2.5 mg
  — 1–3 years 5 mg
  — greater than 3 years 10 mg.
- Paracetamol 15 mg/kg suppository.

🔲 Transport to hospital unless all the following are present:

- Fitting stopped and child fully recovered, and has had similar previous fits due to high temperature alone.
- Temperature returned to normal.
- Parents present and happy to care for child at home.
- Easy access to medical care if fitting recurs.
- Cause of temperature does not require hospital treatment.

HEAT EXHAUSTION

> ⚠ **Temperature over 41°C is immediately life threatening.**

Pathophysiology
- Usually follows exercise.

Assessment/presentation
- Assess for other medical conditions, especially myocardial infarction, diabetes.
- Assess temperature.
- Assess degree of dehydration.

Management
- Ensure ABCDs.
- Administer 60% oxygen.
- ECG monitoring.
- Remove excessive clothing.
- If unconscious:
  - 🔲 immediate evacuation to hospital
  - cold IV fluids en route to hospital
  - 1 litre N/saline STAT.
- If temperature is over 41°C:
  - cool rapidly using fine mist of water
  - ice packs to groins, neck and axillae
  - 🔲 evacuate to hospital
  - alert hospital and advise of possible need for dantrolene (this drug may take them time to find, anaesthetists usually know where it is kept).
- If conscious:
  - remove to cool place
  - give cooled electrolyte solution orally
  - establish IV access
  - give 1 litre N/saline over 30 minutes if unable to take oral fluid.
- Check capillary blood sugar.
- Tepid sponging.
- Check for other causes of hyperthermia, e.g. Ecstasy ingestion.

HYPOTHERMIA

Pathophysiology
- Immersion is major cause.
- Often associated with alcohol ingestion.

Assessment
- ABCDs.
- Respiratory rate may be very slow, as may pulse. Check for at least 1 minute.

Management
- In general, warming should take place at the same speed at which cooling occurred.
- Look for the cause — injury, other illness.

General
- Start Basic Life Support.

 A person is not dead until warm and dead (or the body will not warm despite appropriate treatment).

- Intubation is not contra-indicated in hypothermia and is needed if the patient cannot maintain the airway by other means or if they are impracticable, e.g. when being evacuated.
- Monitor cardiac rhythm, start Advanced Life Support
  - VF may be unresponsive to cardioversion at temperatures below 30°C.
  - Bradycardia is a sign of low metabolic rate and does not require atropine.
  - Most arrhythmias correct as the temperature returns to normal.
  - Many drugs are ineffective at low temperature.
  - Acidosis and hypoxia are the common causes of arrhythmias.
- Most hypothermic patients are hypovolaemic due to the diuresis of vasoconstriction; balance need for fluids with delay in evacuation. Always use warm fluid and ensure it remains warm in tubing.
- Check capillary blood sugar (if low give intravenous dextrose, not glucagon).

Temperature

- Safety of self
    - Keep yourself warm and dry.
    - Do not give your clothes away unless surplus to requirements.
- Avoid further heat loss
    - Remove from cold environment.
    - Protect from wet or cold ground.
    - Wrap in windproof outer layer.
    - Wrap with insulating layers (multiple blankets).
    - Cover the head.
    - Avoid oxygen from a cold cylinder unless vital.
- Rewarm
    - Warm inspired air (use specific warmer if possible).
    - If uninjured and conscious give warm drink and source of carbohydrate, e.g. chocolate.
    - Get into warm ambulance as soon as possible.

Space blankets reflect heat. They will therefore reflect any heat from external sources away from the body. They should only be used if the major heat source is within the space blanket

MENINGITIS / MENINGOCOCCAL SEPTICAEMIA

 Many people with meningitis are initially diagnosed as having flu.

Assessment/presentation

In meningococcal septicaemia, the signs of meningitis are often absent.

- Preceding flu-like illness.
- Vague headache.
- Pyrexia.
- Photophobia.
- Neck stiffness.
- Non-blanching rash (roll a glass over the rash and it does not change colour).

Management

- Ensure ABCDs.
- Administer 60% oxygen.
- Get intravenous access.
- Give 1.8 g benzylpenicillin IV.

 Any delay in giving antibiotics can be fatal.

- If IV access is difficult give penicillin IM initially.
- Give fluid bolus of 1 litre colloid STAT.
- ⬛ Arrange immediate transfer to hospital.
- Before departing, advise contacts to speak to their general practitioner or public health department in next few hours.
- Speak to occupational health if you have had direct contact with secretions.

Alternative antibiotic:

- Cefotaxime.

Early antibiotics save lives.

MYOCARDIAL INFARCTION

In suspected myocardial infarction

- Check ABCs.
- Attach to ECG monitor and treat arrhythmia accordingly.
- Give oxygen, at least 60%.
- Sit patient up, unless severe hypotension.
- Give entonox as initial analgesia.
- Give aspirin 300 mg orally (unless history of allergy).
- Give 1–2 metered doses of glyceryl trinitrate if systolic blood pressure > 100 mmHg.
- Establish IV access.
- Give diamorphine and metoclopramide intravenously. (This not only relieves pain but reduces risk of arrhythmia.)
- Target on scene time of less than 20 minutes.
- Transport to nearest hospital capable of administering thrombolytic therapy. Inform hospital, including presence or absence of contraindications to thrombolysis.
- If no appropriate hospital within 15 minutes' journey time then consider commencing thrombolysis. This requires a 12 lead ECG to confirm the diagnosis.
- Check for contraindications to thrombolysis (see below).

> ⚠ **Only give pre-hospital thrombolysis if you have the ability to deal with any subsequent problems.**

- If none present and appropriate facilities available give:
- Intravenous rTPA bolus and IV heparin bolus.

Contraindications to thrombolysis

- Bleeding disorder.
- Recent surgery (within 2 weeks).
- Previous cerebrovascular accident.
- Active peptic ulceration.
- Possible aortic dissection.
- Traumatic cardiac massage.
- Trauma.
- Diabetic retinopathy.
- Pregnancy.

Every minute's delay to thrombolysis means more dead heart muscle.

NEONATAL RESUSCITATION

Table 2.1
Apgar score

	0	1	2
Pulse	0	1–100	>100
Respiratory effort	nil	slow irregular	strong cry
Muscle tone	absent	flexion	active movement
Colour	all blue	blue limbs	pink
On suction	nil	depressed	coughs well

 Remove all meconium before ventilating.

Management
- Perform Apgar unless obviously distressed.
- Cover the child.
- If meconium in airway, before ventilating:
  — suction of airway
  — intubate but do not ventilate, suction via ET tube, extubate.
- Ventilate with bag and 100% oxygen.
- Give naloxone 10 µg/kg, if mother had opiate.
- If not improving, intubate.
- Ventilate with 100% oxygen.
- Commence cardiac massage.
- Adrenaline 10 µg/kg every 5 minutes.
- Check capillary blood sugar.
- Warm baby.
- 🚑 Transport to hospital.

Most babies are successfully resuscitated with a few minutes' oxygen.

PAEDIATRIC EMERGENCIES

RESUSCITATION

Guidelines for paediatric resuscitation are shown on pp 66–67 (Fig. 2.8).

Basic Life Support

Figure 2.7 illustrates the Resuscitation Council's protocol for Basic Life Support in children.

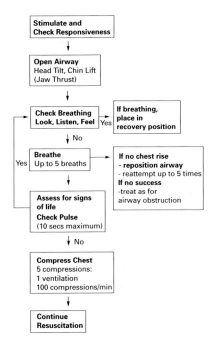

Fig. 2.7   Paediatric Basic Life Support.

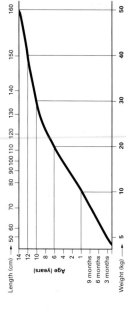

Endotracheal tube

Oral length (cm)	18-21	18	17	16	15	14	13	12	10
Internal diameter (mm)	7.5-8.0 cuffed	7.0 uncuffed	6.5	6.0	5.5	5.0	4.5	4.0/3.5	3.0-3.5

Weight (kg) →	5	10	20	30	40	50
Adrenaline (ml of 1 in 10 000) **initial** intravenous or intraosseous	0.5	1	2	3	4	5
Adrenaline (ml of 1 in 1000) **Subsequent** intravenous or intraosseous (or initial endotracheal)	0.5	1	2	3	4	5
* Atropine (ml of 100 µg/ml) intravenous or intraosseous (or double if endotracheal)	1	2	4	6	6	6
Atropine (ml of 600 µg/ml)	-	0.3	0.7	1	1	1
Bicarbonate (ml of 8.4%) intravenous or intraosseous (dilute to 4.2% in infants)	5	10	20	30	40	50
* Calcium chloride (ml of 10%) intravenous or intraosseous	0.5	1	2	3	4	5

	0.4 / 2.5 mg	0.8 / 5 mg	1.6 / 10 mg	2 / 10 mg	2 / 10 mg	2 / 10 mg
Diazepam (ml of 5mg/ml emulsion) intravenous or rectal / Diazepam (mg rectal tube solution) rectal						
Glucose (ml of 50%) intravenous or intraosseous (dilute to 25% in infants)	5	10	20	30	40	50
* Lignocaine (ml of 1%) intravenous or intraosseous	0.5	1	2	3	4	5
Naloxone neonatal (ml of 20 µg/ml) intravenous or intraosseous	2.5	5	-	-	-	-
Naloxone adult (ml of 400 µg/ml)	-	0.25	0.5	0.75	1	1.25
* Salbutamol (mg nebuliser solution) via nebuliser (dilute to 2.5-5.0 ml in normal saline)	-	2.5 mg	5 mg	5 mg	5 mg	5 mg
Initial DC defibrillation (J) for VF or VT with no pulse	10	20	40	60	80	100
Initial DC cardioversion (J) for SVT with shock (synchronous) or VT with shock (non-synchronous)	5	5	10	15	20	25
Initial fluid bolus in shock (ml) crystalloid of colloid	100	200	400	600	800	1000

*CAUTION! Non-standard drug concentrations may be available:
Use **Atropine** 100 µg/ml or prepare by diluting 1mg to 10 ml or 600 µg to 6 ml in normal saline.
Note that 1 ml of **calcium chloride** 10% is equivalent to 3 ml of **calcium gluconate** 10%.
Use **Lignocaine** (without adrenaline) 1% or give twice the volume of 0.5%. Give half the volume of 2% or dilute appropriately.
Salbutamol may also be given by slow intravenous injection (5µg/kg), but beware of the different concentrations available (eg 50 and 500 µg/ml).

Reproduced by kind permission of P. Oakley

Fig. 2.8 Paediatric resuscitation chart.

Advanced Life Support

Figure 2.9 illustrates the Resuscitation Council's protocol for Advanced Life Support in children.

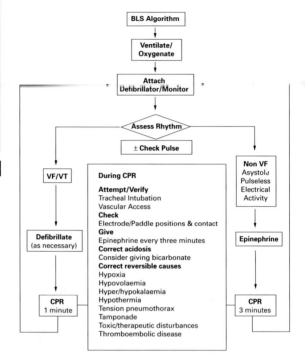

Fig. 2.9 Paediatric Advanced Life Support.

ASSESSMENT OF THE SICK CHILD

Assessment

Airway
- Noises of breathing.
- Large tongue easily obstructs airway.

Breathing
- Work of breathing — use of accessory muscles, positioning, recession.

- Noises — grunting, stridor, wheezing.
- Respiratory rate.
- Ability to speak and drink.

Circulation
- Pulse and blood pressure.
- Capillary refill (in infants, use sole of foot).
- Skin colour and temperature.
- Conscious level (see below).

Disability/conscious level
- Attention to environment.
- Lack of reaction to strangers/procedures.
- AVPU and Glasgow Coma Scale ($\rightarrow$ p 100).
- Posture.

Other
- Temperature.
- Fontanelles.
- Petechial (non-blanching) rash.

Table 2.2 Normal values			
	Pulse	*BP*	*Respiratory rate*
Newborn	160	80/50	60
1 year	120	80/50	40
2 years	110	80/50	30
4–6 years	100	100/70	20
8–10 years	90	110/80	15
12 years	80	120/80	12

Management
- Clear airway.
- Give highest oxygen concentration possible.
- Assisted ventilation if floppy.
- ◪ Move to hospital as matter of urgency.
- Inform hospital.
- 20 ml/kg colloid IV or IO STAT.
- Check blood sugar.
- Give penicillin if any suspicion of meningitis.

The very sick child needs oxygen, volume and a hospital (and possibly penicillin).

BREATHLESS INFANT

Differential diagnosis

- Croup.
- Bronchiolitis.
- Epiglottitis.
- Asthma.
- Choking.

Normal values for respiratory rate

- < 1 year = 30–40
- 1–5 years = 20–30

Management for all cases

- Avoid upsetting the child.
- Let child adopt preferred position — often sitting on parent's lap leaning forward.
- Give oxygen by best tolerated route; letting parent hold tubing near face is often successful.
- Consider nebulised saline.
- ■ Transport to hospital.
- Give specific treatments listed below in the ambulance.

Croup vs. epiglottitis

Croup	Epiglottitis
Gradual onset	Rapid onset
Intermittent stridor	Continuous stridor
Hoarse voice	Snoring-like stridor
Barking cough	Struggles to talk
May be apyrexial	Pyrexial
Can swallow fluids	Drooling

Epiglottitis

- Now rare because of Hib vaccination.
- Life threatening.
- Never examine the mouth or pharynx.
- Rapid transfer to hospital.
- Advise hospital of diagnosis — they should have paediatrician and anaesthetist ready to receive you.
- If child sustains respiratory arrest, consider needle cricothyrotomy.

Croup

- Can be managed at home, unless respiratory distress, difficulty feeding or parental concern.
- Most need oxygen only, en route to hospital.
- Moderate cases show use of accessory muscles, intercostal recession.
- Moderate cases may benefit from nebulised saline.
- Severe cases will show tiredness, rising pulse and high respiratory rate.
- Severe cases:
  — Give nebulised adrenaline 5 ml 1:1000 to buy time.
  — Advise hospital of need for anaesthetist.

Bronchiolitis

- Can be managed at home, unless respiratory distress, difficulty feeding or parental concern.
- Moderate cases show use of accessory muscles, intercostal recession.
- Most need oxygen only en route to hospital.
- Severe cases will show tiredness, rising pulse and high respiratory rate.
- Severe cases need rapid transportation to hospital.

POISONING

Management
- Ensure ABCs.
- Put in recovery position.
- Check capillary blood sugar.
- Consider whether specific antidote is available and either administer or advise hospital of need before arrival.
- Collect all tablets from scene/get list of chemicals at scene.
- Give activated charcoal, except for organic substances and alcohol based substances.
- Do not induce vomiting.
- Keep any specimens of vomit.
- Get advice from National Poisons Information Service 0121 554 3801.

 There are very few specific antidotes.
Most poisonings require supportive treatment.

Antidotes

Poison	Antidote
Opiates	Naloxone
Hydrofluoric acid	Calcium gluconate
Organophosphates	Atropine
Cyanide	Sodium nitrate and sodium thiosulphate
Benzodiazepines	Flumazenil
Hypoglycaemia	Dextrose

Specific overdoses
Aspirin
- Tinnitus, headache, nausea.
- Sweating, tachypnoea.
- Intravenous fluids, charcoal.

Benzodiazepines
- Sedation, respiratory depression.
- ABCs.
- Reverse with flumazenil if unable to support respiration by other means.
- Activated charcoal.

Cyanide
- Metal finishing, house fires.
- Often rapidly fatal.
- 100% oxygen.
- Dicobalt edetate 300 mg IV.
- Sodium thiosulphate 50 ml of 25%.

Iron
- Even small amounts can be fatal.
- Abdominal pain, vomiting.
- Do not give charcoal, as oral antidote will be given in hospital.

Opiates
- Respiratory depression and pin point pupils.
- Support ventilation.
- Naloxone if unable to support ventilation.
- Give IM dose then IV, in case patient responds and runs off.

Organophosphates
- Pesticides.
- Dyspnoea, arrhythmias, bradycardia, muscle twitching.
- Oxygen.
- Atropine 2 mg every 5 minutes until pulse > 80.
- Diazemuls for twitching.

Paracetamol
- Abdominal pain and vomiting.
- Activated charcoal.
- Take to hospital for estimation of blood levels however well patient appears.

Tricyclic antidepressants
- Convulsions, arrhythmias.
- ECG monitoring.
- Activated charcoal.
- Bicarbonate for arrhythmias.
- Diazemuls for fitting.

Volatile agents
- Hallucinations, arrhythmias, anoxic effects.
- ECG monitoring.
- Oxygen.
- May have resistant VF; three shocks then intubate, CPR and transport.

PREGNANCY

HAEMORRHAGE

Principles are the same as for other internal haemorrhage.

Management
- Ensure ABCDs.
- Administer 60% oxygen.
- Put in left lateral position to prevent caval obstruction.
- Transport to hospital.
- Establish IV access.
- Give IV fluids if systolic BP < 100 mmHg.
- Give syntometrine IV for post-partum haemorrhage (PPH) and incomplete miscarriage.

ECLAMPSIA

> Fits due to eclampsia kill 10 women per year.

Assessment/presentation
- Pregnant, in last trimester.
- Health records may show high blood pressure, protein in urine.
- Oedema.
- Fitting.

Warning signs
- Headache.
- Visual disturbance.
- Vomiting.
- Abdominal pain.
- Jitters (hyperreflexia).

Management of fit
- Ensure ABCDs.
- Put in left lateral position.
- Administer 60% oxygen.
- Diazepam 5–10 mg IV.

- Strobe lights and noise can precipitate further fits.
- A good escort may be preferred.
- Take to maternity unit with ITU facility.
- Alert hospital.
- The only true prevention of further fits is delivery.

Management of pre-eclampsia with warning signs

- Give oxygen.
- Check BP.
- Give antacid.
- Lie in left lateral position.
- Establish IV access.
- Transport to hospital. Minimise on scene time.
- A calm, quiet, efficient approach is vital.
- Inform hospital even if only warning signs are present.

If possible, discuss the case with the hospital before transport; ask about giving diazepam prophylactically.

> **⚠ Always keep pregnant women tilted to the left to avoid caval compression.**

PSYCHIATRIC EMERGENCIES

Assessment

Look for organic causes:

- Alcohol or drug abuse.
- Alcohol withdrawal.
- Cerebral malaria.
- Hepatic failure.
- Hypertensive encephalopathy
- Hypoglycaemia.
- Hypoperfusion.
- Hypoxia.
- Puerperal.
- Renal failure.
- Sepsis.
- Thyrotoxicosis.

 In the agitated or confused patient always look for an organic cause.

Mental Health Act

Section 2
- Assessment ± treatment.
- Admission necessary for patient's health or safety of others.
- Valid 28 days.
- Needs approved social worker, one approved psychiatrist and one other doctor.

Section 3
- Admission for treatment.
- Valid six months.
- Specified diagnosis.
- Admission for treatment necessary for patient's health or safety of others.
- Application by approved social worker or nearest relative.
- Needs approved psychiatrist and another doctor.

Section 4
- Emergency admission.
- By approved social worker and any fully registered doctor.
- Duration 72 hours.

Section 135
- Magistrates warrant.
- Requested by approved social worker.
- For self neglect, or protection.

Section 136
- Police officer.
- From public place.
- Duration 72 hours.

Exemption
- Those under influence of alcohol or drugs.

Common law
- Life saving treatment can be given if it is considered that the patient is not in a fit state to understand the dangers of refusing.
- Wishes made when of sound mind must be respected.

 Most psychiatric patients are not aggressive and respond to calm reassuring speech.

Drugs
- Haloperidol IV 5–30 mg.
- Chlorpromazine oral 25–100 mg.
- Diazemuls IV 5–20 mg.
- Lorazepam oral 1–2 mg.

PULMONARY OEDEMA

Assessment/presentation

- May be presentation of acute myocardial infarction. Other causes include severe hypertension, fluid overload, valvular heart disease, and acute arrhythmia.
- Can have non-cardiac causes, e g head injury, inhalation injury, heroin overdose. These cases often need urgent paralysis and ventilation and therefore should be rapidly evacuated to hospital.

- Clammy.
- Distressed.
- Pale.
- Tachycardia.
- Crepitations.
- Gallop rhythm.

Management
- Ensure ABCDs.
- Administer 60% oxygen.
- Sit up with legs dependent.
- Observe pulse, BP, oxygen saturation.
- Apply ECG monitor.
- Establish intravenous access.
- Diamorphine 2.5–5 mg IV with 10 mg metoclopramide.
- Buccal nitrate 3–5 mg providing systolic BP > 100 (or 2 puffs of GTN spray sublingually).
- Frusemide 50 mg IV.
- 🕐 On scene time should not exceed 20 minutes.
- If critically ill should not exceed 10 minutes.
- If not improving, aminophylline 250 µg IV over 20 minutes.

If in critical condition
- Give oxygen.
- Buccal nitrate.
- 🕐 Remove to ambulance if close to patient.
- Give remainder of treatment en route.
- On scene time, 10 minutes.
- Inform hospital.

Section 3

Trauma

PRINCIPLES OF TRAUMA CARE

A Airway control and oxygenation
Spine control

B Breathing and ventilation

C Control of haemorrhage
Circulation

D Disability and neurological assessment

E Environment control

2 Secondary survey only if there is time and patient is not critical

Assessment at scene
- Follow ABCD principle.
- As soon as patient reaches a critical condition, *either*
  — undertake curative action on scene, *or*
  — load and go, continuing treatment en route.

The Golden Hour
- An unproven concept.
- Many trauma victims die before the end of the first hour.
- Time belongs to the patient.
- The patient with serious injuries starts deteriorating from the time of injury.
- If you cannot stop deterioration you may be able to slow it down.
- Make sure time you spend is of benefit to the patient's overall care.

The three most common causes of preventable pre-hospital trauma death
- Failure to control the airway.
- Failure to deliver patient rapidly to someone who can stop haemorrhage (a surgeon).
- Delay with penetrating trauma.

Actions undertaken at scene that may convert critical to non-critical

- Complete relief of obstructed airway.
- Administration of oxygen.
- Relief of tension pneumothorax.
- Ventilation of the comatose patient.
- Control of external haemorrhage.

Actions that are usually best undertaken in hospital

- Insertion of chest drain.
- Treatment of cardiac tamponade.
- Treatment of massive haemothorax.
- Control of internal haemorrhage.

Actions that only buy time until definitive care can be obtained

- Needle cricothyrotomy.
- Any non-cuffed airway control in the comatose.
- Spine control.
- Dressing open pneumothorax.
- Manual stabilisation of flail segment.
- Stabilisation of pelvic fracture.
- Intravenous fluids.
- Limitation of bleeding by splintage.
- Rewarming.
- Cardiopulmonary resuscitation in trauma.

These actions are important but can also delay more important definitive care. Informed decisions need to be made about whether to undertake them at the scene or en route to hospital.

 Critical trauma needs no more than 10 minutes on scene.

MECHANISMS OF INJURY

Certain types of accidents are associated with a spectrum of injuries. Similarly, groups of injuries occur: if one is present, look for another; for convenience these are listed on one line. By specifically looking for these injuries, instead of waiting until they become apparent, fewer will be missed.

Head-on RTA

Impact may be decreased by seatbelts and airbags.

- Head and facial injuries (against windscreen or seat in front of rear seat passenger).
- Neck injury (extension–flexion).
- Closed chest injury, e.g. flail chest, lung contusion, myocardial contusion (chest against steering wheel).
- Patella fracture, femur fracture, pelvis fracture (knee hitting on dashboard).
- Foot injury (from pedals).

Side-impact RTA

Side-impact bar and side airbags may decrease injury.

- Head and neck (intrusion against head).
- Fractured humerus, flail chest (door impact against side of body).
- Fractured pelvis, visceral injury (side intrusion within seat).
- Tibia, foot degloving (footwell compaction).

Motorcyclist frontal impact

- Head and neck injuries (head on to road).
- Fractured humerus, flail chest (impact on road).
- Fractured femur, wrist fracture/dislocations, groin injuries (on handlebars as victim leaves cycle).

Pedestrian hit by car

- Tibia fracture, knee disruption (bumper injury).
- Flail chest (bonnet injury).
- Head and neck injury (roof injury).

Fall from height

- Fractured calcaneum, fractured hip, fractured pelvis, vertebral collapse (fall on feet).
- Head and facial injuries, wrist injuries (fall forward).
- Head, neck, arm, shoulder (head first).

Deceleration injury

Sudden deceleration for whatever reason causes injury at junction of mobile and immobile structures:

- C spine.
- L spine.
- Aortic arch.
- Duodeno-jejunal junction.
- Ileo-caecal junction.
- Brain injury/intracranial haematoma.

TRAUMA

 Airway control takes priority over everything else in trauma, but should be undertaken in conjunction with spine control.

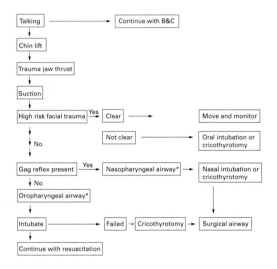

Fig. 3.1 Airway control in trauma (see also p 130).

Whenever cricothyrotomy is undertaken, consider whether conversion to a surgical airway is required, e.g. more than 20 minutes to definitive care, need for cuff to protect airway.

When intubation is indicated, consider the alternative techniques:

- Orotracheal intubation — the gold standard but needs good access.
- Nasotracheal — needs person to be breathing, can be undertaken blind.
- Combitube — can be undertaken completely blind.

Is anaesthesia required to

- Prevent rise in intracranial pressure?
- Prevent vagal stimulation?
- Enable oral intubation?

 All trauma patients need oxygen — use high flow and a mask with a reservoir.

Trauma patients are dying for oxygen.

BURNS — AIRWAY

 The airway is the early killer in burns.

 **The airway deteriorates rapidly.
When stridor occurs it is too late.
Burnt airways need expert anaesthetists.**

☐ Laryngeal and airway oedema develop rapidly. If any high risk features are present, an expert anaesthetist is needed, therefore give oxygen, load and go.

High risk airway
History
- Entrapment in smoke filled room.
- Coughing after evacuation.
- Coughing up black sputum.
- Unconsciousness, even if reversing with oxygen.

Signs
- Respiratory rate > 30.
- Respiratory distress.
- Oedema of lips.
- Burns around mouth.
- Intraoral blisters or soot.
- Singed nasal hair.
- Hoarse voice or stridor or wheezing.

Management

- High flow oxygen.
- ⚑ Transport immediately to nearest A&E with anaesthetic support (do not delay by going to Burns Unit).
- Nebulised salbutamol if wheezing.
- Do not insert any oral or nasal tube.
- Use cricothyrotomy if airway obstruction develops.
- Remember possibility of toxic inhalation, e.g. carbon monoxide, cyanide.

Carbon monoxide poisoning

- Remove from source of carbon monoxide.
- Ensure ABCs.
- 100% oxygen.
- If respiratory rate > 30 or < 10, assist ventilation.
- Beware false high reading of pulse oximeter.
- Continue 100% oxygen however much the patient improves.
- Transport to hospital.

Early intubation is a life saver but can kill in inexperienced hands.

FACIAL INJURY

 Facial injuries should always be considered as a source of airway obstruction — present or developing.

AIRWAY OBSTRUCTION

- Haemorrhage.
- Mechanical obstruction.
- Oedema.

The last, in particular, may develop over time but can usually be predicted from the mechanism of injury.

Management of airway obstruction in facial injury

- Lying the patient supine may be fatal. The patient often controls his own airway by positioning himself to allow drainage and spitting out the blood.
- The person with a facial injury who is talking may be developing airway obstruction that will need surgical control.

- Chin lift and jaw thrust.
- Check for impacted dentures, broken teeth, etc.
- Manual disimpaction of maxillary fracture by grasping the maxilla with the index and middle fingers inside the mouth.
- Pull tongue forward, if necessary grasp with forceps or a suture to secure.
- Suction.
- High concentration of oxygen.
- Lean patient forward or lie prone to allow gravity to drain blood from mouth and nose (but remember that neck cannot be adequately controlled in these positions).

 An informed decision must be made of relative risks to airway and spine.

- Arrest of nasal haemorrhage:
  — Pinch nose for anterior bleeding.
  — Insert nasal tampons if not controlled.
  — Insertion of Foley catheter is not advised in facial
     fractures in the field because of potential malposition.
- Nasopharyngeal airway and nasal intubation are
  contra-indicated.
- If oropharyngeal airway is tolerated then a cuffed tube is
  needed in trachea.
- Oral intubation under direct vision.
- Blind techniques of oral intubation (e.g. Combitube) may
  be difficult.
- Avoid anaesthesia in the field as it may be impossible to
  intubate (the one thing worse than an obstructed airway is
  an obstructed airway in a paralysed patient).
- Needle cricothyrotomy to improve oxygenation.
- Surgical airway to improve oxygenation and ventilation as
  well as protecting the airway with a cuffed tube.

 **High-risk facial injuries should have
airway care and then rapid transportation.**

MANAGEMENT

The only major components of pre-hospital management of
facial injury are the control of the airway and associated
haemorrhage control.

- Airway control as described above.
- Cervical spine control — the mechanism of blunt facial
  trauma invariably carries a high risk for cervical spine injury.
- Breathing is not usually compromised by isolated facial
  injury.
- Aspirated teeth can cause lower airway obstruction.
- Circulation often has to be controlled as part of airway
  control.
- External haemorrhage can usually be controlled by direct
  pressure.
- If foreign body is present leave in situ and press around
  area with a circle of gauze.
- Never explore wounds of face or neck.
- Bleeding tooth socket can be controlled by biting on a
  gauze roll placed over the socket.

> ⚠️ **The spine must be presumed to be injured until proven otherwise. This may be a clinical decision but more often requires radiological support.**

- Check ABCs.
- **A** Immobilise the spine whilst undertaking airway manoeuvres.
- Continue immobilisation.

IMMOBILISATION OF C SPINE

There are only two correct ways of immobilising the cervical spine.

1. Manual immobilisation
- Holding the head does not immobilise the spine unless the shoulders are also immobilised.
- Several techniques are available:
  — From in front, hold side of head in hands and rest forearms on patient's chest.
  — From side, one hand on chin with that forearm on chest, other hand on back of head with that forearm resting on upper back.
  — From behind, hold side of head in hands and rest forearms on back of shoulders.
  — From behind in supine position, place thumbs on collar bones and touch finger tips together over upper thoracic spine whilst gripping the head between the forearms.

2. Collar, side support and tape
- A collar alone is inadequate immobilisation.
- The patient must be lying down or have the full length of the supine strapped to an immobiliser to ensure adequate immobilisation.

> ➤ The immobilisation of the spine should
> continue whilst other resuscitation is
> undertaken. It is often most appropriate to continue
> manual immobilisation whilst ABCs are treated.
> An appropriate bystander can often undertake this.
>
> It is better to delay application of the collar, side
> supports and tape than to delay essential ABC
> resuscitation.
>
> The only exception to these rules is the agitated
> patient (e.g. children, drunks, and restless head
> injuries). In these cases suboptimal manual
> immobilisation or a hard collar may be all that can
> be achieved, and some immobilisation is better
> than none.
>
> Do not forcibly restrain the patient; it is assault
> and may cause more damage. Resisting against
> immobilisation puts greater stress on a fracture/
> dislocation than does ordinary unresisted
> movement.
>
> See extrication techniques (pp. 91–93) for
> techniques of whole spine immobilisation.

- **B** Assess adequacy of ventilation.
- Look for abdominal breathing.
- Give supplemental oxygen.
- Assist ventilation if respiratory rate < 10 or > 30 or
  decreased oxygen saturation.

C Treat for hypovolaemia in first instance.

Neurogenic shock
- Associated with injury above T6.
- Sympathetic nervous supply damage.
- Features:
  — hypotension
  — vasodilatation
  — bradycardia.
- Treatment:
  — Ensure ABCs corrected.
  — Trendelenburg position (but observe for respiratory
    distress and avoid in head injury).

— One litre of intravenous fluid.
— 0.5 mg atropine IV.

Always look for other causes of shock before diagnosing neurogenic shock.

SPINAL INJURY — NOT IMMOBILISING

Patients who do not require spinal immobilisation after injury — satisfy all these criteria

- Fully conscious and orientated.
- No complaint of central neck pain or back pain.
- No neurological symptoms (e.g. numbness, pins and needles, weakness).
- No tenderness over spinous processes of spine.
- No neurological signs.
- No distracting painful injuries.
- Can appreciate pain (alcohol, drugs, analgesia; age; mental state).
- No high risk mechanism of injury.

High risk accidents

- Ejection from a vehicle.
- Roll over RTAs.
- Motorcyclist with helmet damage.
- Pedestrian/cyclist thrown by accident.
- Diving, rugby, horse riding, gymnastics.

EXTRICATION

All these techniques presume adequate immobilisation of the C spine (→ pp. 89–91).

 Spinal immobilisation is important BUT it can also be a major cause of delay in transferring the critically injured patient to hospital.

Patient supine

- Scoop stretcher transfer.
- Vacuum mattress.

Patient prone

Either

- Log roll to 90°.
- Apply spinal board to back.
- Roll onto spinal board in supine position.

Or

- Scoop under patient.
- Spinal board against his back.
- Strap board to scoop.
- Roll through 180°.
- Remove scoop.

Patient in vehicle — critical injuries

- Insert spinal board from side under patient's buttock.
- Rotate patient so back is to board, with minimum of rotation of spine.
- Bring board up against patient's back.
- Lower board and patient to horizontal position.
- Slide patient along board.
- Secure on board.

Patient in vehicle — non-critical injuries

Method one

- Support patient in position and slightly lower seat back.
- Insert extrication device behind patient (this may require roof removal).
- Secure extrication device to patient.
- Fasten leg straps.
- *Either* lift patient in device.
- *Or* slide out on spinal board in the extrication device.
- Place on vacuum mattress.
- Remove extrication device, unless less than 15 minutes' journey to hospital.

Method two

- Lower seat back whilst supporting patient (if hatchback, lower patient until board can be inserted through tailgate).
- Insert backboard against patient (may require roof removal if not hatchback).
- Lay patient against backboard.
- Tilt board to horizontal position if possible.
- Slide patient along spinal board.
- Secure patient to board.

If time on board will exceed 30 minutes, then transfer on to a vacuum mattress using a scoop stretcher.

HELMET REMOVAL

It is better to control the patient's airway with his helmet on and remove it at a later stage. The helmet can be taped down or held by a bystander whilst you resuscitate.

Leave open face helmets in situ. Check whether the face component can be opened (it often has two red buttons on the side to allow this).

Technique
- Rescuer one stabilises the helmet.
- Rescuer two immobilises neck by supporting mandible with thumbs, passing fingers around back of neck and resting forearms on clavicles.
- Rescuer one inserts fingers inside the sides of helmet and pulls it open by lateral traction.
- Rescuer one slides helmet beyond the occipital protuberance.
- Rescuer two slides fingers up to occipital protuberance.
- Rescuer one slides front of helmet past nose.
- Rescuer one slides helmet off.
- Rescuer one takes over manual immobilisation of the spine.
- Take helmet to hospital to demonstrate damage.

VENTILATORY PROBLEMS AND CHEST TRAUMA

Pathophysiology

There are six immediately life-threatening problems that need to be considered in assessing the chest in the primary survey:

1. Airway obstruction.
2. Tension pneumothorax.
3. Massive haemothorax.
4. Open pneumothorax.
5. Flail chest.
6. Cardiac tamponade.

 All those with respiratory distress need oxygen and pulse oximetry and may need assisted ventilation.

General principles

- Patients are best transported in semi-erect position; need informed decision if possibility of spinal injury.
- All need oxygen and pulse oximetry.
- If respiratory rate >30 or <10 then assist ventilation.
- Pain relief before transport in the non-critical will improve ventilation.
- Haemoptysis indicates significant lung injury.
- If patient is unconscious, tilt spinal board with injury side lowermost to improve ventilation and stop aspiration of blood into uninjured lung.

Tension pneumothorax

Features

- Often develops after penetrating trauma or in ventilated trauma patients.
- Rapidly deteriorating respiratory distress.
- Raised jugular venous pressure (JVP).
- Tracheal deviation, hyper-resonant chest, decreased breath sounds ipsilaterally.

Management
- Oxygen.
- Pulse oximetry.
- Rapid needle decompression.
- ▣ Rapid evacuation to hospital.
- Chest drain usually best delayed until arrival at hospital.

Massive haemothorax
Features
- Respiratory distress.
- Dull percussion to chest.
- Decreased air entry.
- Hypovolaemic shock.

Management
- Oxygen.
- Pulse oximetry.
- ▣ Transport to hospital.
- IV infusion.
- Insert chest drain only if prolonged transfer time; risk of releasing tamponade.

Open pneumothorax
Features
- Wound (may be hidden at back).
- Presume all chest wounds are deep if they go through the skin.
- Respiratory distress.
- Resonant percussion note.
- Decreased breath sounds.

Management
- Do not remove any weapon.
- Oxygen.
- Pulse oximetry.
- Dressing with flutter valve.
- ▣ Transport.
- Observe for developing tension pneumothorax.
- If tension pneumothorax develops, treat as above or remove dressing and insert finger in wound.

Flail chest

There are two elements to this injury:

- Flail segment causing ventilatory difficulty.
- Damage to underlying lung.

Cardiac contusion is also possible.

Features
- Side-impact RTA.
- Segment moving paradoxically.
- Surgical emphysema.
- Associated pneumothorax.
- Haemoptysis.

Management
- Oxygen.
- Pulse oximetry.
- Analgesia (not Entonox).
- Stabilisation of chest wall (manual pressure or strapping until arrival in hospital).
- ECG monitoring.
- ◼ Transport to hospital.

Cardiac tamponade

Usually results from penetrating chest trauma.

Features
- Raised JVP.
- Hypotension.
- Muffled heart sounds.
- May only develop after initial fluid bolus.

Management
- ◼ Immediate transport as most important treatment is thoracotomy.
- Oxygen.
- Pulse oximetry.
- ECG monitoring.
- If rapidly deteriorating, pericardiocentesis may buy some time.

Other chest injuries may need treatment but are not usually as time dependent.

Cardiac contusion

Usually results from blunt chest trauma.

Features
- Often asymptomatic.
- Hypotension caused by heart failure.

Management
- Oxygen.
- Pulse oximetry.
- ECG monitoring.
- Most arrhythmias need correction of hypoxia only.
- Only treat arrhythmias if symptomatic.

Rib fractures and chest wall contusion

Feature
Pain on breathing.

Management
- Oxygen.
- Pulse oximetry.
- ECG monitoring.
- Pain relief (not Entonox).

Getting oxygen in is easier than getting carbon dioxide out.

CIRCULATION AND HAEMORRHAGE CONTROL

The emphasis in the treatment of hypovolaemic shock is now changing. Until recently, aggressive pre-hospital fluid resuscitation was advocated. Now controlled hypotension is becoming the accepted pre-hospital treatment. The rationale is:

- Blood is best replaced with blood, which is not available on scene.
- Haemorrhage should be controlled before restoring the blood pressure.
- Surgery is required for internal haemorrhage, not fluid.
- Raising blood pressure may restart bleeding.
- Coagulopathy may follow excessive fluid resuscitation.
- Fluid overload is detrimental, especially in head and chest injury.

Estimating fluid loss
- Visual assessment of external loss.
- Assessment of vital signs.

Blood loss	Pulse	BP	Respiratory rate
< 750 ml	< 100	Normal	14–20
750–1500 ml	> 100	↓pulse pressure	20–30
1500–2000 ml	> 120	↓ systolic BP	30–40
> 2000 ml	> 140	very low	40+

Known injury patterns:

- Pelvis 2000 ml.
- Femur 1000 ml.
- Tibia 750 ml.

 Haemorrhage control is more important than fluid replacement.

Haemorrhage control
Massive blood loss occurs from 5 sites:

- Chest.
- Abdomen.

- Pelvis.
- External injuries.
- Multiple major limb fractures.

Control of haemorrhage can be achieved in the following ways:

- Chest — needs surgery.
- Abdomen — needs surgery.
- Pelvis:
  — Close pelvic ring and immobilise by strapping, extrication device, pneumatic anti-shock garment (PASG), vacuum mattress.
  — Urgent transport to hospital for external fixation.
- External injuries:
  — Simple pressure.
  — Elevation.
  — Temporary suturing of wound.
  — Clips/tourniquet only as last resort.
- Limb fractures:
  — Traction splintage of fractured femur.
  — Vacuum splintage of other limb fractures.

Fluid resuscitation

- Commence after control of haemorrhage or en route to hospital.
- Target systolic BP 100 mmHg.
- Fluids should be warmed.
- Hartmann's is preferred initial fluid.

Vascular access

- Peripheral venous access.
- Femoral venous access.
- External jugular access.
- Venous cutdown.
- Intraosseous infusion.

These are discussed in Section 5 ($\rightarrow$ p 129).

Hypotension in pregnancy

Always consider hypotension caused by vena caval obstruction.

- Manually displace uterus to left.
- Tilt patient to left on a spinal board.

> *Filling up a tank does no good if there is still a hole in it.*

ASSESSMENT

Assess ABCs first

History
- Mechanism of injury, including energy involved and localisation of any force.
- Protective helmets and damage to them.
- Loss of consciousness, fits.
- Amnesia.
- Any neurological symptoms.
- Co-existing medical conditions, medication.
- Alcohol, drug history.

D Examination — primary survey

AVPU
- **A**lert and responding to command.
- **V**ocal stimulus before responds.
- **P**ainful stimulus required to produce response.
- **U**nresponsive.

Pupils
- Size.
- Equality of size.
- Reaction to light.
- Evidence of local injury (this may affect response and is a common reason for a fixed dilated pupil).

Glasgow Coma Scale

 4. Eyes; 5. mouth; 6. limbs.

Eyes
1. No response
2. Responds to pain only
3. Responds to vocal command
4. Opens eyes spontaneously

Verbal (details in brackets are paediatric variations)
1. No verbal response
2. Incomprehensible noises (irritable, inconsolable)
3. Words but inappropriate (moaning)

4. Confused speech (consolable)
5. Normal conversation

Motor
1. No movement
2. Extends limb (stretching) to painful stimulus
3. Flexes limb (curls up) to painful stimulus
4. Withdraws from pain
5. Localises to source of pain
6. Moves limbs to command

< 8 = Severe head injury
9–12 = Serious
13+ Minor head injury at present

 Minor head injuries can deteriorate with time. They need careful assessment (→ p 102).

MAJOR HEAD INJURY

Management
- Airway control:
  — Avoid stimulating gag reflex causing rise in intracranial pressure.
  — Pulse oximetry.
  — High flow oxygen.
- Spine control:
  — Presume cervical spine injury in any unconscious patient.
- Ventilation:
  — Paralyse and ventilate to maintain normal/low carbon dioxide levels.
- Circulation:
  — Hypotension is not due to head injury.
  — Maintain systolic BP at approximately 100 mmHg.
  — Avoid fluid overload.
- D — intracranial pressure:
  — Anaesthesia and paralysis avoids increases in ICP.
  — Mannitol can buy time if patient is rapidly deteriorating, but discuss with local neurosurgeons.

Good head injury care is simply attention to ABCDs.

MINOR HEAD INJURY

A head injury can only be called minor after the patient has
fully recovered. Even the fully conscious patient can develop
long-term problems such as post-concussion syndrome and
psychological disorders.

This section deals with the person who is fully conscious
and alert on arrival of the emergency services.

Does this person need to attend hospital?

A person can be allowed home from the scene only if all the
following conditions apply:

- No loss of consciousness at any time.
- No amnesia.
- No fits.
- No neurological signs and symptoms.
- No evidence of basal skull fracture (CSF or blood from
  ears, nose or mouth; bilateral black eyes, mastoid bruising).
- No scalp haematoma.
- No full thickness scalp laceration.
- No alcohol intoxication.
- You are able to fully assess the person (i.e. not confused,
  postictal, very young, etc.).
- Absence of complicating co-existing medical disorders.
- Mechanism of injury is not high risk (e.g. high-energy
  accident, localised trauma). High-risk injuries include those
  such as from golf balls, baseball bats, objects falling from a
  height.

The patient must also be given appropriate advice about
seeking help and be accompanied by a responsible adult for
the next 24 hours.

Management

All other patients should be taken to hospital for assessment.

- Ensure ABCDs.
- Determine whether spinal immobilisation is required.
- Check for external wounds and dress appropriately.
- Check pupils.
- Calculate Glasgow Coma Score (→ p 100).
- Look for abnormal neurology.
- Record the above findings every 15 minutes en route to
  hospital.

Principles
- Usually part of secondary survey.
- May be part of haemorrhage control, i.e. 'C'.
- Immobilise injury site and joint above and below.
- Check distal circulation.
- Check distal sensation.

Early reduction reduces pain and complications.

> **No fracture is trivial to the victim, they all cause pain. Remember, Sir Robert Peel died of complications of a fractured clavicle (subclavian vessel tear).**

Pre-hospital treatment
Remember, slings are only effective when the patient is semi-erect or sitting up. If a collar and cuff is too painful, then use a broad arm sling.

All soft tissue injuries and fractures benefit from:

- Immobilisation
- Pain relief
- Elevation
- Local ice.

Table   Limb support in trauma

Injury	Support	Risks
Sterno-clavicular dislocation	Posterior is critical trauma	
	Anterior — support with broad arm sling	
Clavicle (fracture)	Broad arm sling	
Acromio-clavicular dislocation	Broad arm sling	
Dislocated shoulder	Patient supporting weight of arm	
Neck of humerus (fracture)	Collar and cuff	
Shaft of humerus	Vacuum splint + broad arm sling	Risk of radial nerve injury
Supracondylar fracture	Vacuum splint + broad arm sling	Risk to brachial artery
Dislocated elbow	Self support or vacuum splint	
Forearm fracture	Vacuum splint	
Wrist fracture	Broad arm sling	
Fractures in hand	High arm sling	
Hip dislocation	Support in presenting position with blankets	Risk to sciatic nerve
Fractured neck of femur	Strap to other leg	
Fractured shaft of femur	Traction splint	Risk to popliteal vessels
Supracondylar fracture of femur	Vacuum splint	
Tibial fracture	Vacuum splint	
Patellar dislocation	Vacuum splint	Reduce on scene if possible
Dislocated knee	Vacuum splint	Risk of neurovascular injury
Ankle fractures	Vacuum splint	
Ankle dislocation	Vacuum splint	Vascular compromise
Foot fractures	Elevate in vacuum splint	

PAEDIATRIC TRAUMA SCORE

Summate the coded values for the six parameters. This gives
a score with a maximum value of 12.

Weight	> 20 kg	+2
	10–19 kg	+1
	< 10 kg	−1
Airway	Normal	+2
	Simple airway	+1
	Intubated/cricothyrotomy	−1
Systolic BP	90 mmHg	+2
	50–89 mmHg	+1
	< 50 mmHg	−1
Conscious level	Awake	+2
	Drowsy	+1
	Comatose	−1
Open wound	None	+2
	Minor	+1
	Major	−1
Fractures	None	+2
	Closed	+1
	Open	−1

NON-ACCIDENTAL INJURY (NAI)

Always consider NAI in every child who is injured. The elderly and those with learning disabilities are also liable to NAI.

> **Every carer has a responsibility to be aware of his or her local child protection procedures and to institute these if there is a suspicion of abuse.**

Suspect NAI if

- Delay in presentation.
- History not consistent with injuries.
- Lack of appropriate parental concern.
- Attempts to avoid detection.
- Changing history.
- Differing histories by different individuals.
- Direct story of abuse from patient.
- Injuries of varying ages.
- Certain injuries are highly suggestive of NAI:
  — tear of frenulum of tongue
  — cigarette burns
  — perineal injury
  — imprint injuries.

It is not the job of the pre-hospital care worker to judge whether NAI has occurred, the suspicion is sufficient to warrant contacting the duty social worker.

Many cases of suspected NAI are cases of poor parenting. These parents also benefit from support that can be provided by the community paediatric team.

All suspected cases should either be taken to hospital or the community team should attend before you leave the scene.

> **Document all your findings with great care. Include quotes from relevant people.**

There is no greater tragedy than the NAI that is repeated because a carer ignored the earlier warning signs.

> ⚠️ **Always check for possibility of airway burns**
> (→ pp. 85–86).

Assessment
- Nature of burning agent.
- Length of exposure.
- First aid undertaken.
- Area burnt (see Fig. 3.2). Patient's palm = 1% body surface area (BSA).
- Depth of burn. This does not affect pre-hospital care except that circumferential full thickness burns can cause constriction.

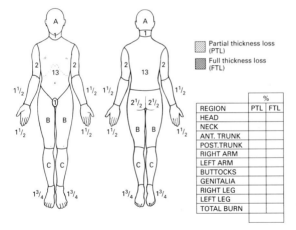

Lund and Browder chart
Ignore simple erythema

Partial thickness loss (PTL)

Full thickness loss (FTL)

REGION	PTL	FTL
HEAD		
NECK		
ANT. TRUNK		
POST.TRUNK		
RIGHT ARM		
LEFT ARM		
BUTTOCKS		
GENITALIA		
RIGHT LEG		
LEFT LEG		
TOTAL BURN		

Relative percentage of body surface area affected by growth:

Area	0	1	5	10	15	Adult
A = 1/2 of head	$9^{1}/_{2}$	$8^{1}/_{2}$	$6^{1}/_{2}$	$5^{1}/_{2}$	$4^{1}/_{2}$	$3^{1}/_{2}$
B = 1/2 of thigh	$2^{3}/_{4}$	$3^{1}/_{4}$	4	$4^{1}/_{2}$	$4^{1}/_{2}$	$4^{3}/_{4}$
C = 1/2 of leg	$2^{1}/_{2}$	$2^{1}/_{2}$	$2^{3}/_{4}$	3	$3^{1}/_{4}$	$3^{1}/_{2}$

Fig. 3.2 Estimation of burn site.

- Is other injury likely?
  — Escaping from building, e.g. jump from height.
  — Explosion, e.g. blast injury or secondary impact.

Management
- Safety
  — Yourself. Is source of burn removed or controlled?
  — Your patient. Has burning agent been removed including drenching with cold water followed by removal of clothes?
  — The scene. Is further burning likely and are fire brigade present?
- Ensure ABCs.
- Airway (→ Burns airway, pp. 85–86).
- Breathing and ventilation
  — If ventilation impaired by circumferential chest burns, undertake escharotomy.
  — Think of toxic substances such as carbon monoxide, cyanide.
  — ■ Transport to hospital and continue treatment en route.
- Circulation — systemic
  — Establish IV access if transit time more than 15 minutes or already hypovolaemic.
  — If hypovolaemic in first 30 minutes, look for other injuries.
  — Calculate fluid requirements. Volume of colloid to be given by 4 hours after burn = (%BSA burnt) × (weight in kg) ÷ 2.
- Circulation — local
  — Check circulation distal to burn.
  — If impaired:
    ◆ elevate limb
    ◆ if circumferential full thickness burn then undertake escharotomy longitudinally, down to bleeding tissue.
- Analgesia
  — Entonox is effective but should not be used if patient was in explosion (risk of pneumothorax) or has inhalational injury (oxygen concentration only 50%).
- Dressing
  — Cover with sterile sheet, or
  — Cover with cling film.

Special considerations

Electrical. See electrocution (p 56).

Chemical

- Safety; protect yourself with protective clothing, including gloves and eye protection.
- Look for Hazchem signs ($\rightarrow$ pp. 6, 7 & 8) and other sources of information.
- Brush off any dry chemical.
- Wash off remaining dry powder or liquid with large amounts of water.
- Irrigate eyes with at least one litre saline via IV giving set.

Special chemical situations

- Hydrofluoric acid
  - Irrigate thoroughly.
  - Apply calcium gluconate gel.
  - If fits, give calcium gluconate IV.
- Alkalis
  - Brush off residue.
  - Use copious amounts of water as reaction with water gives off heat.
- Alkali metals, e.g. sodium, potassium
  - Keep covered with oil.
  - Water will cause explosion.
- Phosphorus
  - Keep immersed under water as burns on exposure to air.
- Phenol
  - If available, wash off with polyethylene glycol.
  - If not available, irrigate copiously with water (small volumes assist absorption of phenol).

Radiation

- The fire service will usually take charge and advise on safety.
- Principles are same as for chemical burns.
- Washing with soap and water is usually sufficient.
- Unless critical trauma, decontaminate at scene.
- Contact hospital before leaving scene — there are designated hospitals for receipt of radiation contaminated patients.

The medical management of the trapped trauma patient is no different from that for any other trauma victim. More prolonged care may be needed at the scene. Interventions usually undertaken in hospital may have to be undertaken at the scene.

Management of the entrapment incident

- Assess the incident
  - Hazards?
  - How many casualties?
  - How many trapped? Absolute (physical) or relative (combination of injury plus physical).
  - How trapped?
- Ensure life saving treatment is underway.
- Adequacy of resources.
- Number of ambulances to transport.
- Appropriate personnel, e.g. need for immediate care doctor/anaesthetist.
- Inform control.
- Liaise with police and fire services.
- Determine exact entrapping forces and components.
- Determine best means of release considering:
  - alternative extrication techniques
  - alternative vehicle cutting, e.g. roof removal, side removal
  - use of analgesia/anaesthesia.
- Continuously monitor progress and patient condition.
- Avoid unnecessary delays.
- Plan evacuation in advance, e.g. helicopter, police escort.
- Keep ambulance control and hospital advised.

Team work of all services is the key to rapid extrication.

CRUSH INJURY

> ⚠️ **Release of a prolonged crush injury can be fatal if incorrectly managed.**

Pathophysiology
- May be caused by:
  — roller type injury over whole limb
  — localised compression with distal ischaemia
  — entrapment with distal ischaemia
  — prolonged use of tourniquet/tight dressing.
- Raised pressure in compartment due to swelling vs. constriction (external or fascial).
- Venous congestion causes swelling which raises pressure causing arterial compression.
- Poor perfusion causes tissue damage with lactic acidosis and release of toxic metabolites, including potassium.
- Reperfusion may cause release of these substances.
- Hyperkalaemia may cause cardiac arrest.
- Myoglobinuria may cause renal failure.

Assessment
- History is the key to diagnosis.
- May be little external evidence.
- May be evidence of decreased perfusion, e.g. loss of pulse, increased capillary refill.
- Skin mottling is a late sign.
- Pain on stretching muscles.

Management
- Ensure ABCs.
- Establish IV access.
- Commence IV Hartmann's infusion.
- ECG monitoring.
- Give analgesia before release.
- Decide if amputation is required
  — Very prolonged ischaemia with non-viable limb.
  — To allow rapid extrication from life threatening environment, e.g. building on fire.

- Decide when to release constriction. If poor perfusion present for more than 30 minutes then:
  — Best to give at least 1 litre Hartmann's before release.
  — Have fast running drip running at time of release.
  — If prolonged ischaemia, consider giving sodium bicarbonate 25 ml 8.4%.
  — If severely ischaemic, consider rapid infusion of dextrose/insulin or calcium gluconate at time of release, to counteract hyperkalaemia.
- Elevate limb as soon as possible.
- Protect limb from injury.

Pathophysiology

- There may be only a small amount of bleeding, this may be caused by:
  — vascular spasm
  — extensive blood loss causing hypotension.
- It may be possible to re-implant the limb.

Management

- Ensure ABCs.
- Arrest haemorrhage.
  — Direct pressure.
  — Elevation.
  — Clips only if above measures fail (clips damage vessels that may be anastomosed later).
  — Tourniquet (but remember the time limit of 60 minutes).
- Fluid replacement (en route to hospital if possible).
- Wash off any gross contamination of severed limb.
- Wrap in gauze.
- Wrap in a plastic bag.
- Put plastic bag in container of iced water if possible.
- Send limb to same hospital as patient (if patient still trapped send limb in advance, so it can be cleaned and stored appropriately).

Assessment of whether limb can be re-implanted

The following will not be suitable

- Severe crushing injury.
- Massive bone or soft tissue loss.
- Other massive life threatening injuries that will take precedence over re-implantation.
- Severe intercurrent illness/fitness for major surgery.

It is best to presume that a limb can be re-implanted and discuss with the receiving surgeon.

PENETRATING TRAUMA TO TRUNK

> **Priorities of medical treatment are the same — ABC.**

> **Penetrating trauma victims can deteriorate very rapidly and then require immediate surgery.**

Management
- Assess safety. Check with police. See firearms incidents (pp. 9–10).
- Never remove penetrating objects.
  — If object is trapping patient, cut well clear of the body.
  — If cutting penetrating object be aware that vibration may start catastrophic bleeding.
  — Ketamine anaesthesia is often indicated for impalement injury.
- Airway control.
- If penetrating trauma to airway or vicinity, MOVE immediately, even if patient is talking.
- Breathing
  — Give oxygen.
  — Needle thoracocentesis for tension pneumothorax.
  — Three sided dressing or dressing with valve over wound.
  — No chest drain for haemothorax as may be tamponading pleural blood.
- Haemorrhage control — apply dressing and pressure.
- Alert hospital.
- Establish IV line en route.
- Give fluids if systolic BP < 90 mmHg.

> **Many firearm and stabbing incidents are drug related. Be prepared for consequences of drug ingestion as well as of the trauma.**

All penetrating trauma to the trunk is serious and needs immediate evacuation to a surgeon.

TRIAGE REVISED TRAUMA SCORE

Summate the coded values for the three parameters. This gives
a score with a maximum value of 12.

Respiratory rate

10–29	4
> 29	3
6–9	2
1–5	1
0	0

Systolic BP

> 90	4
76–89	3
50–75	2
1–49	1
0	0

Glasgow Coma Scale (→ p 100)

13–15	4
9–12	3
6–8	2
4–5	1
3	0

 **If any of the parameters does not score 4 this
indicates serious injury.**

A score of:

- < 10 indicates approximately 25% mortality.
- < 6 indicates greater than 50% mortality.

Problems with scoring system

- Up to 20% of serious injuries may be underscored.
- Not accurate for children or very old.
- Not accurate for pregnant women.
- Head injuries may be underscored.
- Does not accurately predict mortality for individual cases.

> ⚠️ **Inform the hospital in any case where a team is required or critical time may be saved by avoiding delay after arrival.**

If possible, direct speech contact with the receiving unit will decrease errors and allow clarification. A standard format:

- ensures nothing is missed
- allows easy interpretation.

Indications for trauma team call

Mechanism of injury
- Fall > 6 metres (or 3 × child's height).
- Other occupant fatality.
- Ejected from vehicle.
- Intrusion into cockpit > 0.5 metre.
- Extrication time > 20 minutes.
- Child hit by car.
- Pedestrian thrown by vehicle.

Injuries
- Continuing airway problem.
- More than one long bone fracture.
- Penetrating trunk injury.
- Disrupted pelvic ring.
- Burns > 15% BSA (or 10% in a child).

Physiology
- Respiratory rate > 29/min.
- Pulse > 130/min.
- Pulse < 50/min.
- Systolic BP < 90 mmHg.
- Glasgow Coma Score < 13.

Content of message
- Age, male/female.
- Type of incident and time of incident.
- History = mechanism of injury.
- Suspected diagnosis.
- Status of ABCDs.

- Active problems and treatment/interventions undertaken.
- Current status, e.g. improving, deteriorating.
- Requirements at hospital.
- Estimated time of arrival.

> **➤ Call early with initial information and then update. At night a hospital may want to call staff in from home which often takes 15 minutes.**

All radio messages must be augmented by a concise verbal handover, which should be in the same format. Written records should be complete before leaving the hospital.

> *The golden hour belongs to the patient. Good communication avoids wasted time.*

TRAUMA — LOAD AND GO

> ⚠ When the situation requires emergency
> hospital treatment within minutes, on scene
> assessment and treatment should stop and be
> continued in the moving ambulance.

Load and go situations

The patient must be assessed and treated in the usual ABCD
order. As soon as any of these conditions is encountered then
on scene treatment should stop and the patient's journey to
hospital be commenced.

- Failure to control airway in the field.
- The obstructing airway in the conscious patient
  (e.g. burns airway, laryngeal oedema).
- Traumatic cardiac arrest.
- Tension pneumothorax.
- Massive haemothorax.
- Cardiac tamponade.
- Flail chest with respiratory compromise.
- Penetrating trunk or neck trauma.
- Hypovolaemic shock from internal haemorrhage.
- Hypovolaemic shock with uncontrolled external
  haemorrhage.
- Head injury with deteriorating Glasgow Coma Score.
- Head injury Glasgow Coma Score < 8 and unable to
  intubate.

> ➤ The only exceptions to these rules are in
> entrapment or difficult evacuation. In this
> scenario, the circumstances should be reported to
> control.

> ➤ Appropriate experienced assistance, e.g.
> immediate care doctor or hospital flying
> squad, should be requested whenever it is not
> possible to load and go.

Section 4

Multiple casualty situation

119

The following information is required for a major incident. The initial report should be made to ambulance control within minutes of arrival at the scene and should be subsequently updated. The information required can be remembered using the pneumonic ETHANE.

START message by stating 'INCIDENT REPORT Inform duty officer. Long message…'.

E xact location
- Exact location in a road giving house number or obvious landmark.
- Ordnance Survey grid reference.

T ype of incident
- Road Traffic Accident involving cars/coaches/lorries — give numbers.
- Rail.
- Air crash.
- Terrorist incident.

H azards present or potential
- Fire.
- Chemical.
- Electricity.
- Biohazard.
- Unexploded device.

A ccess to the incident
- Give accurate direction of approach from nearest main road.
- Request that police be informed of this route.
- Will ambulance service need different approach to other services?
- Think of the circuit for access and egress and a parking point.
- Detail a reporting point for all health service staff arriving at the scene.

Number of casualties and severity

- Initially state number of walking wounded and number of stretcher cases.
- Later give more details including approximation of severity of injuries and number trapped.
- Details of type of injuries if possible, e.g. burns, spinal, glass injuries.

Emergency services, present and required

- Detail of services that can be seen on site.
- Detail further ambulance/medical resources required.
- Do you need:
  — BASICS doctors
  — hospital team
  — specialist rescue, e.g. cave rescue
  — local authority
  — military including bomb disposal
  — coastguard
  — commercial, e.g. chemical advice, tanker owners?

END message by stating 'DECLARE MAJOR INCIDENT — xx.xx hrs. CONFIRM'.

MAJOR INCIDENT — FIRST ON THE SCENE

If you manage nothing else, declare a Major Incident and give an ETHANE report.

- Park in a safe location close to the incident, not stopping the traffic flow.
- If you have an assistant, leave him in the vehicle as the initial control point.
- Leave beacons on, to mark control point.
- Don protective clothing and tabard.
- Carry out a rapid reconnaissance.
- Declare Major Incident.
- Give ETHANE report (→ pp. 120–122).
- Determine special resources required:
  — Major Incident support vehicle
  — Off road vehicles
  — BASICS doctors
  — Hospital medical team.
- Work out route for approach and exit of ambulances.
- Look for site for casualty clearing station.
- Prepare briefing for Ambulance Incident Officer.
- Continue task of AIO (→ p 123) until his arrival.

AMBULANCE/MEDICAL INCIDENT OFFICER CHECKLIST

- Park your vehicle in a safe place. Leave keys with police.
- Put on protective clothing and identification tabard.
- Find Ambulance Incident Officer if present and work together.
- Confirm your presence with ambulance control, and confirm your callsign.
- Ensure that triage is underway.
- Ensure that only Priority One patients are being brought from incident.
- Ensure that walking wounded have a collecting point.
- Find Fire and Police Incident Officers.
- Recheck ETHANE ($\rightarrow$ p 120–121).
- Establish more accurate casualty numbers.
- Decide on route of ambulance flow.
- Decide on resources needed:
  — ambulances
  — ambulance personnel
  — immediate care doctors
  — hospital teams
  — first aiders, Voluntary Aid Society (VAS)
  — Forward Incident Officer.
- Decide location of:
  — casualty clearing station and triage point at entry
  — ambulance parking point
  — ambulance loading point
  — temporary mortuary.
- Mark out the appropriate areas.
- Inform hospitals of situation.
- Find out availability and limitations of hospitals in area.
- Brief staff as they arrive.
- Keep a log of all events.
- Record all staff sent forward and give them a time to return to control vehicle.
- Arrange rest periods.
- Plan for continuing staff needs.
- Consider use of other transport (e.g. buses) for walking wounded and arrange appropriate hospital reception.
- Arrange regular meetings of all Incident Officers.
- Appoint Safety Officer.
- Arrange regular checking of stock levels at scene.

STAFF BRIEFING — ON ARRIVAL AT MAJOR INCIDENT

 All staff should be briefed on arrival at scene to ensure maximum efficiency.

- Introduce AIO and MIO.
- Describe incident:
  — exact location of incident relative to briefing point
  — type of incident
  — hazards
  — access to incident and overall geography
  — number of casualties
  — emergency services present.
- Location of:
  — emergency control vehicle
  — casualty clearing station.
- Describe command and control structure.
- **All tasks must be authorised by Incident Officer.**
- **At end of each job, return to Incident Officer.**
- Communications
  — Describe on scene communications.
  — Remind that only Control Vehicle and Incident Officers speak to Ambulance Control.
  — State call signs of key individuals.
- Give out individual tasks.
- Time staff due back for a break.
- Time of next briefing.
- Ask for questions.

TRIAGE SIEVE

- Rapid assessment taking only a few seconds.
- Sieve and then move to next patient.
- Someone else should follow to evacuate or treat Priority One patients.
- Walking wounded can be instructed to walk to a pre-arranged collecting point.

Can the patient walk?
- Yes → Priority 3 (Green). Tell to walk to collecting point for P3
- No → Proceed with sieve

Is the patient breathing?
- No, even after airway opened → Dead (or ALS only if sufficient resources)
- Yes, after airway manoeuvre → Priority 1 (Red)
- Yes, without airway manoeuvre → Proceed with sieve

What is respiratory rate?
- Over 30 per minute → Priority 1 (Red)
- Under 10 per minute → Priority 1 (Red)
- 10–30 per minute → Proceed with sieve

What is circulatory status?
- Capillary refill greater than 2 seconds → Priority 1 (Red)
- Capillary refill under 2 seconds → Priority 2 (Yellow)

Move to next patient.

Exceptions

The sieve is only a guide. There are exceptions who will be undertriaged by this system and it is then appropriate to re-grade them.

- Children have different physiological norms.
- Burns may be life threatening but patient may be walking.
- Chemically contaminated patients may need urgent decontamination.
- Extensive bleeding, that will deteriorate if not stopped.

Aim is to do most good for the most people within your limited resources.

There may be several field triage officers initially. Each will work in a defined geographical area.

- Only take on this role on instruction of AIO.
- Ensure you have supply of triage labels and oral airways.
- Check location of CCS and walking wounded area.
- Check you know the geographical area you have been asked to cover.
- Undertake triage sieve (→ p 125).
- Your only treatment is simple airway control.
- Use bystanders to control airway if needed.
- Ensure that only Priority One patients are moved initially.
- Keep a count of how many cards of each priority you have issued.
- When triage in your area complete return to AIO.
- Inform of number of casualties and triage code.
- Ask for further instructions.

TRIAGE OFFICER AT CASUALTY CLEARING STATION ENTRANCE

- Check on field triage code.
- Repeat triage sieve.
- Check all patients entering CCS are triaged and labelled.
- Ensure that distinct areas exist for each triage category.
- Arrange priority one patients in two areas:
  — those requiring immediate treatment
    (nearest CCS entrance)
  — those requiring immediate evacuation
    (nearest ambulance loading point).
- Keep count of each category as they enter CCS.
- If possible record ID number of all those entering CCS.
- Keep Incident Officer informed of numbers. Initially report back every 15 minutes to AIO.

MASS GATHERING CHECKLIST

PLANNING

- Does major incident plan exist for location?
  — Who would be AIO/MIO?
  — Where is casualty clearing station?
  — Where is ambulance route, parking point, loading point?
  — Are staff aware of their role?
  — Are other emergency services aware of this plan?
  — Are stewards, site security fully briefed for major incident?
- What specific problems may occur with this type of event?
- Get information from similar events.
- Liaise with police regarding potential problems.
- Decide numbers of first aiders, technicians, paramedics, and doctors.
- Decide location of field hospital and first aid posts.
- Define communications system between medical services, to ambulance control, to organisers, to police, to local A&E.
- Refreshments organised for staff.

Day before
- Local A&E aware.
- Ambulance control aware.
- Meet with organisers and police.
- All personnel confirmed attendance.
- Check equipment inventory.

On the day
- Brief all staff.
- Talk to local A&E Sister.
- Talk to ambulance control.
- Make one person responsible for staff breaks and refreshments.
- After one hour check with staff that no problems have arisen.

End of the day
- Check with police and organisers before standing down staff.
- Debrief and thank all staff.
- Write report including lessons learnt for next time.

Section 5

Procedures

129

Oropharyngeal airway

Advantages
- Simple.
- Widely available.

Disadvantages
- Induces vomiting.
- Does not protect airway from aspiration.
- Possible damage to teeth during insertion.
- Easily dislodged if manual support not continued.

Insertion technique
- Select correct size of airway:
  — length of airway = distance from angle of jaw to corner of mouth
  — average adult = size 3.
- Open mouth.
- Insert in inverted position.
- When tip is past back of tongue, turn through 180°.
- Close mouth around airway.
- Support chin.

Nasopharyngeal airway

Advantages
- Can be inserted in presence of clenched jaw.
- Tolerated in the semi-conscious.
- Does not induce vomiting.

Disadvantage. Can cause epistaxis.

Contra-indications
- Nasal trauma.
- Epistaxis.
- Basal skull fracture.

Insertion technique
- Select correct size of airway:
  — should easily pass through nares
  — adult female = 6, adult male = 7.
- Insert large safety pin through flange to prevent it sliding inside nose.
- Lubricate well.
- Gently slide tube along floor of nasal cavity.

AIRWAY FORMULAE

 Do not guess. Always check important formulae. Have one size above and below ready.

	Formula	Average adult male	Average adult female
Oropharyngeal airway	—	4	3
(*Quick technique* Length = corner of mouth to ear)			
Nasopharyngeal airway	—	7	6
(*Quick technique* Diameter = internal diameter of nares)			
Laryngeal mask airway	—	4	3
Orotracheal tube size	(age/4) + 4	9	8
Orotracheal tube length	(age/2) + 12	23 cm at teeth	21 cm at teeth
Nasotracheal tube size	(age/4) + 3	8 cm	7 cm
Nasotracheal tube length	(age/2) + 15	26 cm	24 cm

Indications
- After initial intubation.
- After moving patient.
- Difficulty ventilating patient.
- Abnormal noises from ET tube or airway.
- Increase in ventilatory pressures.

> **Risk of tube displacement is decreased by:**
> - **taping tube securely**
> - **use of semi-rigid collar**
> - **briefly disconnecting during transfers from stretcher to bed, etc.**

Checks
- See tube passing through the vocal cords.
- Auscultation of breath sounds in both axillae but not in epigastrium.
- Misting of tube with each breath.
- Ability to aspirate 50 ml of air via the tube.
- Maintenance of normal oxygen saturation.
- Fluctuating end tidal CO_2 level.
- Improving colour of patient.

NEEDLE CRICOTHYROTOMY

Indications
- Emergency airway control when
  - simple adjuncts failed
  - definitive airway not possible
    - ◆ urgency of situation
    - ◆ trismus or gag present.

Contraindications
- Trauma to anterior neck.
- Surgical emphysema/inability to determine local anatomy.
- Need for airway protection, i.e. cuffed tube.

Equipment
- 12 gauge venous cannula or specific needle cricothyrotomy needle.
- 10 ml syringe.
- Y connector or 2 ml syringe.
- Oxygen supply and tubing.

Procedure
- Locate cricothyroid membrane (Fig. 5.1).
- Place thumb and index finger either side of cricothyroid membrane to stabilise the cricoid and put tension on the skin.

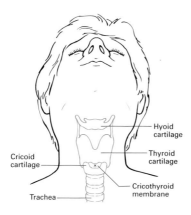

Fig. 5.1 Anatomical landmarks for needle and surgical cricothryrotomy.

- Insert cannula through skin and cricothyroid membrane at 45° caudally.
- Aspirate through 10 ml syringe as advancing needle, until air is aspirated.
- Slide cannula into trachea over stylet.
- Remove syringe and stylet.
- Connect to Y connector.
- Connect oxygen supply at 12–15 litres/min.
- To insufflate, occlude side port for one second, leave open for 4 seconds.
- Arrange for definitive airway within 20 minutes.
- Secure in place but do not bend tube by attaching on to skin.

Alternatives. If no Y connector is available, a side port can be cut in the oxygen tubing. This is inserted and secured in the barrel of a 2 ml syringe and connected to the cannula.

SURGICAL CRICOTHYROTOMY

Indications
- Emergency airway control when
  — simple adjuncts failed
  — oro/nasotracheal intubation not possible
    ◆ facial injuries
    ◆ lack of anaesthesia
    ◆ personal experience of carer.

Contraindications
- Children under 12 years (immature cartilage rings).
- Trauma to anterior neck.
- Surgical emphysema/inability to determine local anatomy.

Equipment
- Local anaesthetic.
- 6 mm tracheostomy tube.
- Securing tape.
- Bag valve mask ventilation system.

Procedure
- Locate cricothyroid membrane ($\rightarrow$ p 133).
- Insert local anaesthetic if required.
- Place thumb and index finger either side of cricothyroid membrane to stabilise the cricoid and put tension on the skin.
- Make a 2 cm transverse incision in the skin and cricothyroid membrane.
- Insert forceps in incision before withdrawing scalpel.
- Open forceps.
- Insert 6 mm cuffed tracheostomy tube (or other cuffed tube).
- Remove forceps.
- Inflate cuff.
- Check that bilateral lung inflation occurs.
- Continue ventilating.
- Secure tube.
- Continue resuscitation.

PULSE OXIMETER

A non-invasive measure of haemoglobin's saturation with oxygen.

Difficulties with pulse oximetry

- Measures saturation not total oxygen carried, therefore a high reading in anaemia may reflect low total oxygen.
- Cannot differentiate carboxyhaemoglobin; a high reading may reflect a large amount of carbon monoxide rather than oxygen.
- Does not reflect ventilation, i.e. carbon dioxide levels may be very high with normal saturation, especially if giving supplemental oxygen.
- Low reading may be due to poor peripheral circulation.★
- Artefact from fluorescent or flickering lights.★
- Movement artefact, including shivering.★
- Some colours of nail varnish may give false reading.

★ These may be detected in those oximeters giving a waveform reading.

Normal values

95–100% — normal when breathing air.
90–95% — represents mild hypoxia when breathing air.
< 90% — represents severe hypoxia if on supplemental oxygen.

 Normal values of oxygen saturation are not a reason for withholding oxygen treatment.

Procedures
Pulse oximeter

136

LOG ROLL

Indications
Any patient with potential spinal injury.

- To insert spinal board behind him.
- To avoid aspiration during vomiting or bleeding in airway.
- To remove objects underneath casualty, e.g. glass.

Procedure (Fig. 5.2)
- One person supports the head and neck.
- Three others place themselves along one side.
- Hand positions are as follows (numbering from head end in order):
  1. tip of shoulder
  2. lower rib cage, inside the arm
  3. pelvis
  4. supporting upper thigh
  5. supporting upper knee
  6. supporting upper ankle.
- Person supporting head is team leader and gives clear commands.
- Gently roll to 90°, pulling towards the rollers.
- Return to position on command of leader.
- Remove hands in reverse of above numerical order.

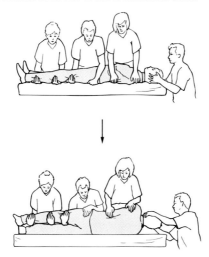

Fig. 5.2 'Log roll'.

NEEDLE THORACOCENTESIS

Indication
Suspected tension pneumothorax.

> ⚠ **This is an emergency procedure and speed is vital.**

Equipment
- Alcohol wipe.
- Intravenous cannula (12 G).
- 10 ml syringe.

Procedure (Fig. 5.3)
- Ensure patient is receiving high flow oxygen.
- Locate second intercostal space (below rib at level of manubrio-sternal junction).
- Locate point at mid-clavicular line in second intercostal space.
- Wipe skin with alcohol swab.
- Insert a 12 G cannula at right angles to skin and advance into pleural cavity.
- Aspirate on syringe as advancing.
- If pneumothorax is present, air will be aspirated.

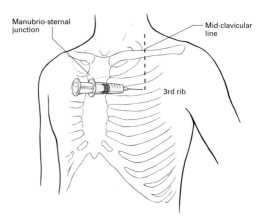

Fig. 5.3 Anatomical landmarks in needle thoracocentesis.

- Remove syringe and stylet.
- Tape cannula in situ ensuring it does not kink at skin entry point.
- If no air is aspirated, remove stylet and syringe in case cannula is blocked with blood or skin plug.
- If still no air release or clinical improvement, remove cannula.
- Tape over wound.
- Make sure receiving unit is told of the procedure.

Aftercare
- Transport to hospital immediately.
- Continue monitoring the patient
- Continue to give high flow oxygen.
- If condition deteriorates without specific cause, presume tension pneumothorax has recurred.

> **This patient will need a chest drain soon, either at hospital or in the field ($\to$ p 151).**

END TIDAL CARBON DIOXIDE (ET CO_2) MONITORING

Uses
- Detection of oesophageal intubation.
- Detection of disconnection or leakage in ventilation system.
- Monitoring of respiration rate and adequacy.
- Rapid detection in changes in cardiac output.
- Monitoring adequacy of CPR.

Difficulties with ET CO_2
- Increases may be due to decreased ventilation, increased perfusion of previously ischaemic tissue or decreased cardiac output.
- Present portable machines are fragile.

> ⚠️ **It is vital that you are familiar with the operation of your defibrillator before you need to use it. Every second's delay decreases the chance of successful cardioversion.**

Indications
- Ventricular fibrillation.
- Pulseless ventricular tachycardia.
- Asystole where VF cannot be excluded.

Contraindications
- Patient is in pool of water.
- On aircraft unless machine approved for use.
- In presence of combustible/ explosive materials, e.g. petrol.

Procedure
Every operator must be fully conversant with his machine. Machines vary in their details but the following rules apply to all:

- Dry the chest before applying gel pads.
- Administer oxygen whilst preparing to check, but do not let oxygen accumulate under sheets, clothing, etc.
- Remove any medication patches from the chest.
- Check for pacemaker, if present use biaxillary shock.
- Select energy level
- Charge up with paddles on chest.
- Shout 'stand clear' before defibrillating.
- Check that no one is in contact with patient before defibrillating.
- Keep paddles on patient between shock 1/2 and 2/3.
- Never take charged paddles off the chest, discharge first.

VENOUS CUTDOWN

Indications
- Venous access by standard routes not possible, and
- Necessity for fluid before arrival at hospital.

Contraindications
- Proximal trauma to the limb.
- Procedure causes inappropriate delay in transport.
- Sepsis around cutdown site.

Equipment
- Scalpel.
- 2 pairs mosquito forceps.
- Suture
- 12 G intravenous cannula.

Sites
- Long saphenous vein
  — 2 cm anterior and superior to the medial malleolus.
- Median cephalic vein
  — 2 cm proximal and lateral to medial epicondyle of elbow.

Procedure
- Clean skin.
- Make a 2 cm incision over the vein (Fig. 5.4).
- Spread subcutaneous tissues longitudinally and identify vein.
- Using blunt dissection, insert forceps behind vein and mobilise.

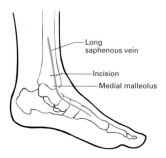

Fig. 5.4 Anatomical landmarks in saphenous vein cutdown.

- Ensure that nerve is separate from vein.
- Having passed forceps around vein, pull 2 sutures back behind the vein.
- Separate the sutures and tie the distal one around the vein.
- Use the proximal one to draw vein out of wound.
- Make a small incision in anterior wall of vein.
- Insert cannula into vein.
- Tie proximal suture around cannula and vein.
- Commence IV infusion.
- If time allows, suture skin, and suture cannula in place.
- Firmly tape cannula and giving set.

PNEUMATIC ANTI-SHOCK GARMENT (PASG)

In the UK, a PASG is a second line treatment except in fractured pelvis. It should only be used to buy time.

Indications
- Hypovolaemic shock due to fractured pelvis.
- Sudden hypotension following release from crush injury.
- Hypovolaemia related to multiple limb fractures.
- Abdominal aortic aneurysm.
- Other causes of hypovolaemic shock, septic shock, anaphylactic shock or neurogenic shock, when other means of control are not possible.

Contraindications
- Chest trauma.
- Severe head injury.
- Pregnancy (relative).
- Compartment syndrome or limb ischaemia.

Disadvantages

> **Studies have shown an increased mortality following PASG application, probably due to the pulmonary complications.**

In inexperienced hands, PASG can delay evacuation to hospital.

Procedure — inflation
- Lay the PASG on a flat surface, e.g. a spinal board.
- Remove sharp objects from patient's pockets, clothing, etc.
- Lay patient on top of PASG.
- Check for contra-indications and recheck that peripheral pulses are present.
- Secure each compartment firmly around limbs and abdomen by the Velcro strips.
- Inflate the leg compartments first, using inflation pressures of 40–60 mmHg.
- Inflate the abdominal component (unless patient pregnant, evisceration, open abdominal injury, diaphragmatic injury).

Procedure — deflation

 Should usually be performed in hospital; must have facilities to transfuse and undertake surgical intervention rapidly on deflation.

- Check that systolic BP > 100 mmHg.
- Ensure two large bore cannulae in situ and working, connected to appropriate fluid.
- Continuously monitor pulse and BP.
- Slowly deflate abdominal compartment.
- If BP falls or pulse rises then increase fluid infusion and stop deflation.
- Undo straps on abdominal component and release.
- Release one leg compartment, monitoring pulse and BP.
- Release other leg compartment with same precautions.
- Undo straps on leg components and release
- Carefully examine limbs and check circulation to limbs.

INTRAOSSEOUS INFUSION

> ➤ **The intraosseous route can be used to administer all resuscitation fluids and drugs.**

Indications
- Need for emergency fluid or drug administration in child under 6 years.
- Inability or expected inability to cannulate peripheral vein.

Contraindications
- Fracture of major bone in that limb.
- Pelvic fracture if using lower limbs.
- Severe soft tissue injury in that limb.
- Previous IO needle in that bone.
- Local sepsis at entry site.
- Osteoporosis, rickets, osteogenesis imperfecta, other bone abnormalities.

Equipment
- Intraosseous needle unthreaded.
- 2 ml syringe.
- Gauze roll and tape.

Sites
- Proximal tibia (Fig. 5.5)
  — at least 2.5 cm below the tibial tuberosity
  — the preferred site.
- Distal femur
  — at least 2.5 cm above line drawn between superior edges of femoral condyles.
- Proximal humerus
  — at least 2.5 cm below the neck of the humerus.
- Medial malleolus
  — 1 cm proximal to medial malleolus
  — the only site that may be consistently suitable for drug administration in adults.

Procedure
- Identify landmarks.
- Clean skin.
- Insert local anaesthetic down to periosteum.
- Insert needle through skin down to periosteum, at 90° to the skin. If necessary make a small skin incision.

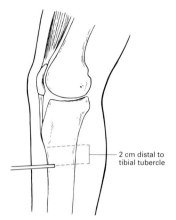

2 cm distal to
tibial tubercle

Fig. 5.5 Anatomical landmarks in femoral nerve block.

- Using a twisting action advance the needle through the bone cortex until a give is felt.
- If a second give is felt the needle has probably gone out of the far side of the bone.
- Check needle is in correct position
  — Flick needle and it should not wobble.
  — Aspirate with 2 ml syringe and marrow should be obtained (save for cross matching).
  — Inject 20 ml saline, which should inject with slight resistance but no swelling of soft tissues.
- Connect to three way tap and giving set.
- Use side port of three way tap to administer fluids or drugs.
- For fluids, aspirate from giving set and then switch tap position and inject into IO needle. Gravity is very slow and this technique is very simple. Also use 20 ml syringe as volume infused = 20 ml/kg, i.e. one syringeful per kg.
- Secure needle using gauze roll either side and plenty of tape in a cruciform dressing.

Complications

- Osteomyelitis (incidence very low if removed within 24 hours).
- Compartment syndrome/tissue injury, from infusion outside marrow cavity.
- Growth plate injury.

FEMORAL NERVE BLOCK

Indication
Fractured shaft of femur.

Contraindications
- Local sepsis or tissue injury in groin.
- Time critical injuries requiring immediate evacuation.

Equipment
- 20 ml syringe.
- 1% lignocaine.
- 0.5% marcaine.

Procedure
- Ensure ABCs secure and IV fluid commenced.
- Mix 10 ml 1% lignocaine and 10 ml 0.5% marcaine in a 20 ml syringe.
- Palpate the femoral artery.
- Insert needle below the inguinal ligament and 1 cm lateral to femoral artery (Fig. 5.6).
- Aspirate to ensure artery not punctured.
- Instil local anaesthetic.
- Repeat procedure so a fan shape of anaesthesia is inserted.
- Anaesthesia should follow in 5–10 minutes.
- Apply traction splint.

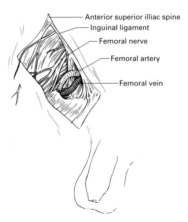

Fig. 5.6 Anatomical landmarks in femoral nerve block.

FEMORAL VEIN CANNULATION

> ➘ This procedure is easily undertaken in the back of a moving ambulance. Rapid fluid volume infusion can therefore be commenced without delaying transfer to definitive care.

Indications
- Inability to obtain venous access by peripheral route.
- Profound hypovolaemia needing pre-hospital infusion.
- Need for venous access for drug administration.

Contraindications
- Local trauma to groin.
- Suspected pelvic fracture.
- When it will cause unacceptable delay in transfer to hospital.

Equipment
- As for peripheral cannulation.
- If possible, use a 6 gauge intravenous cannula.
- Gauze roll and tape.

Procedure
- Clean the skin.
- Palpate the femoral artery.
- Insert cannula through skin 1 cm medial to femoral artery.
- Direct cannula at 45° to the skin, pointing towards head.
- Aspirate continuously until venous blood aspirated.
- Advance cannula over needle.
- If unsuccessful, move slightly laterally and attempt again.
- If you enter femoral artery, remove cannula and apply firm pressure for 10 minutes.
- If possible, take a 10 ml sample of blood for the hospital to use for cross match.
- Connect to fluids and giving set.
- Secure in place — it is best to rest the protruding cannula on a gauze roll so that it does not kink at the skin entry point.

See diagram of femoral triangle in description of femoral nerve block (p 148).

INSERTION OF CHEST DRAIN

> ⚠ **Insertion of a chest drain in the field is a difficult procedure with increased mortality and morbidity over in-hospital insertion. Careful consideration must be given to whether it would be safer to evacuate the patient rapidly and then perform the insertion.**

Indications
- Tension pneumothorax after needle decompression.
- Massive haemothorax.
- Open pneumothorax.

AND

- Recurrent tension despite needle thoracocentesis.
- Prolonged entrapment.
- Long journey to hospital.
- Aeromedical evacuation.

Contraindications
- Close proximity to hospital relative to time to undertake procedure.
- Patient's condition is stable.
- Suspected haemothorax without intravenous access.

Equipment
- Chest drain: size 30/32 Fg for an adult; child (age + 10) Fg. Discard the trocar.
- Skin preparation, e.g. alcohol swab.
- Local anaesthetic.
- Scalpel, large dissecting forceps.
- Drainage system with valve.
- Suture, securing tape.

Procedure
- Ensure patient is receiving high flow oxygen.
- Locate fifth intercostal space in mid-axillary line.
- Lift patient's arm to shoulder level and get someone to support it there.
- Clean the skin and infiltrate local anaesthetic, all the way down to pleura.

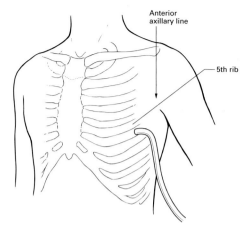

Fig. 5.7 Anatomical landmarks for inserting a chest drain.

- Make a 4 cm incision through skin and subcutaneous tissues, just above 6th rib.
- Insert dissecting forceps through intercostal muscles directly above 6th rib and split muscles horizontally.
- Pierce pleura with finger or closed forceps.
- Slide finger along forceps and into pleural cavity.
- Sweep finger around to ensure no adhesions.
- Grasp end of chest tube with forceps and slide along finger to introduce it into the pleural cavity towards the apex of the lung.
- Attach drainage bag with one-way valve.
- Suture the wound.
- Secure the tube (most easily done by wrapping adhesive tape around the tube and suturing tape to skin).
- There is no need to insert a purse string suture at this stage.
- Apply waterproof tape over tube and insertion site.

Aftercare

- Monitor patient's condition, including pulse oximetry.
- ◪ Transport to hospital as soon as possible.
- Continue high flow oxygen.

Section 6

Drugs

> ⬊ The drugs stocked will vary according to the training of the individual and the type of pre-hospital care work being undertaken. A more extensive formulary would be required for those undertaking mass gathering medicine.

Adenosine	Frusemide
Adrenaline (epinephrine)	Glucagon
Aminophylline	Glyceryl trinitrate spray
Aspirin	Haloperidol
Atropine	Hydrocortisone
Benzylpenicillin	Ipratropium
Buccal nitrate	Lignocaine
Charcoal	Metoclopramide
Chlorpheniramine	Naloxone
Chlorpromazine	Paracetamol
Dextrose injection	Paraldehyde
Dextrose gel 40%	Prednisolone
Diamorphine	Salbutamol injection
Diazepam rectal	Salbutamol nebuliser
Diazemuls	solution
Flumazenil	Syntometrine

Anaesthetic agents are discussed on pp. 157–159. They are not considered appropriate for most pre-hospital carers.

STORAGE OF DRUGS

Temperature

All drugs have specific storage requirements. Most drugs will
not tolerate the high temperatures experienced in the boot of
a vehicle in summer. Some drugs need cold storage. Special
refrigeration facilities are available for use in vehicles.

Controlled drugs

- A register must be kept of all Schedule One and Two
  controlled drugs.
- Records of when drugs are used, destroyed or disposed of
  must be kept in this book, as must details of drugs currently
  in store.
- Each drug must be listed on a separate page.
- Entries must be clear, legible and indelible.
- The record must be kept for seven years after the last drug
  is used.
- Schedule One and Two drugs must be stored in a double
  locked container.
- A locked container in a vehicle is only allowable if the
  vehicle is locked.
- A locked glove box is not considered adequate.

For details of specific drugs see pp. 160–169.

Timing
- After primary survey.
- May be part of 'B' — to help adequate ventilation.
- To aid extrication/evacuation.
- Must not delay transportation of critical patient.

Methods
- Psychological
  - Reassurance is a powerful reliever of pain.
- Splintage
  - Stopping fracture movement reduces pain with minimal side effects.
- Inhalational
  - Rapidly and easily given.
  - Not for use in divers, head or chest injury.
- Regional anaesthesia
  - Good analgesia with minimal side effects.
  - Takes time to work.
  - Difficult in pre-hospital care.
- Parenteral analgesia
  - In the seriously ill, the intravenous route is preferred.
  - Opiates are usually the best agents.
  - Titrate dose to effect.
- Anaesthesia
  - Provides complete anaesthesia.
  - Proven benefit in head injuries.
  - Can speed up extrication.
  - Needs experience.

Storage
→ p 155.

Indications

- After primary survey in most circumstances.
- To aid extrication/evacuation.
- Must not delay transportation of critical patient.
- May be part of 'A' if cannot control/protect airway otherwise.
- May be part of 'B' to improve ventilation.
- Improves outcome in head injury by improving oxygenation and ventilation and averting rises in ICP.

Monitoring

It is vital to have adequate monitoring in place during anaesthesia. This should ideally be automated.

- ECG.
- Pulse oximeter.
- NIBP every 5 minutes max.
- End tidal carbon dioxide if intubated (ideal but not essential).

What is required for personnel undertaking anaesthesia in the field?

- Adequate training.
- Adequate number of cases per year.
- Continuing training.

 Presume that every patient has a full stomach.

Technique

- Prepare equipment.
- Establish monitoring.
- Pre-oxygenate if possible.
- Establish IV access and give fluid bolus.
- Ensure adequate space and access.
- Lay out equipment in accessible location.
- Have at least two assistants, one of whom should know the equipment.
- Mix your own drugs and label syringes.
- Cricoid pressure.
- Anaesthetise.

Anaesthetic agents

Emergency pre-hospital use requires intravenous agents.

Ketamine
- Can be used for analgesia or dissociative anaesthesia.
- Not for use in head injuries, eye injuries, hypertensive patients.
- Combine with midazolam to decrease risk of emergence hallucinations.
- Does not suppress respiration, elevates blood pressure.
- May not suppress gag reflex, therefore intubation may not be possible.
- Dose: 0.5–2 mg/kg.

Thiopentone
- Do not use until volume restored, can cause sudden severe hypotension.
- Ideal for brain injury.
- Slowly metabolised, redistributed quickly; therefore anaesthesia wears off but hangover effect.
- Stored as powder.
- Dose: 3–5 mg/kg (6–7 mg/kg in children).
- Beware extravasation and intra-arterial injection.

Propofol
- May cause hypotension.
- Short acting as rapidly metabolised.
- Avoid in egg allergy and elderly.
- Dose: 2 mg/kg.

Etomidate
- Causes less hypotension.
- Dose 100–300 µg/kg per minute.

Muscle relaxants

Suxamethonium
- Quick acting, short lasting.
- Second dose should be preceded by atropine.
- Chloride needs storing in fridge; bromide is a powder for reconstitution.
- Do not use in burns.
- Dose: 0.6 mg/kg

Vecuronium

- Good in shocked patient.
- Powder form.
- Long acting — 30 minutes.
- Dose: 80–100 µg/kg bolus then 20–30 µg/kg as required.

Atracurium

- Degrades, therefore unaffected by renal or hepatic blood flow.
- Good in shocked patients.
- Dose-dependent duration.
- Avoid in asthma.
- Needs storage in fridge.
- Bolus 300–500 µg/kg.

Only those with appropriate training and experience should undertake anaesthesia in the field.

The information contained in this section is an aide memoire. It does not replace texts such as the British National Formulary. It does not aim to be exhaustive in its description of drugs.

Drug doses are for a healthy 70 kg adult unless otherwise stated.

Adenosine

Indication	Supraventricular tachycardia
Dose	Rapid infusion of 3 mg, 6 mg, 12 mg incrementally until effect Infuse into large vein and flush immediately
Contraindications/ caution	2nd or 3rd degree heart block, asthma, heart transplant Must have continuous monitoring

Adrenaline

Indication	Cardiac arrest, anaphylaxis
Dose	10 ml of 1:10 000 for cardiac arrest 1 ml of 1:1000 intramuscularly (or subcutaneously) for anaphylaxis *CHILD 10 μg/kg initially then 100 μg/kg IV or IO for cardiac arrest*
Contraindications/ caution	None in cardiac emergencies

Aminophylline

Indication	Reversible severe bronchospasm
Dose	5 mg/kg over 20 minutes
Contraindications/ caution	Patients already taking oral preparation should not receive this Risk of cardiac arrhythmia, fits

Aspirin

Indication	Myocardial infarction
Dose	150 mg p.o.
Contraindications/ caution	Not for use in children Hypersensitivity

Atropine

Indication	Asystole, bradycardia
Dose	Asystole 3 mg IV once Bradycardia 300–1000 µg IV
	Organophosphate poisoning 2 mg IV every 20 minutes until responds *CHILD Asystole 20 µg/kg, minimum 100 µg*
Contraindications/ caution	None in cardiac emergencies

Benzylpenicillin

Indication	Suspected meningitis or meningococcal septicaemia
Dose	1.2 g IV or IM *INFANT 300 mg* *CHILD 1–9 years 600 mg*
Contraindications/ caution	Hypersensitivity Give IM if delay in giving IV

Buccal nitrate

Indication	LVF
Dose	2–5 mg retained in buccal sulcus
Contraindications/ caution	Hypotension, hypersensitivity to nitrates May cause headaches, dizziness, postural hypotension

Charcoal (activated)

Indication	Poisoning with absorbable agents when no oral antidote to be given
Dose	50 g orally
Contraindications/ caution	Absent or diminished gag reflex, dysphagia

Chlorpheniramine

Indication	Anaphylaxis
Dose	10 mg IV
Contraindications/ caution	Transient hypotension, urinary retention, glaucoma, hepatic disease

Chlorpromazine

Indication	Agitation, hyperthermia
Dose	25–50 mg by deep IM injection
Contraindications/ caution	Phaeochromocytoma Postural hypotension, hypothermia

Dextrose 50% solution

Indication	Hypoglycaemia
Dose	25–50 ml until clinical improvement *CHILD 2 ml/kg of 25% solution*
Contraindications/ caution	Use large vein and flush after use

Dextrose 40% gel

Indication	Hypoglycaemia
Dose	20–50 ml
Contraindications/ caution	Must be able to protect own airway

Diamorphine

Indication	Pain relief, LVF
Dose	2.5–10 mg IV slowly, according to effect *CHILD 0.05–1 mg/kg*
Contraindications/ caution	Use with care in head injury or patients with decreased conscious level Have naloxone available

Diazepam rectal

Indication	Persisting fits
Dose	*CHILD 1–3 years 5 mg; > 3 years 10 mg*
Contraindications/ caution	Respiratory depression or insufficiency, hepatic impairment

Diazemuls

Indication	Prolonged fits
Dose	10–40 mg IV *CHILD 0.25–0.5 mg/kg IV*
Contraindications/ caution	Respiratory depression or insufficiency, hepatic impairment

Flumazenil

Indication	Respiratory suppression caused by benzodiazepines
Dose	200 µg, then 100 µg every minute up to 1 mg
Contraindications/ caution	Epileptics on benzodiazepine treatment Occasionally causes fits

Frusemide

Indication	Pulmonary oedema
Dose	50–100 mg IV
Contraindications/ caution	Liver failure, anuria Can cause hypotension

Glucagon

Indication	Hypoglycaemia, unless prolonged or alcoholic
Dose	1 mg IM or IV
Contraindications/ caution	Secreting tumours Give oral glucose on recovery

Glyceryl trinitrate

Indication	Angina, LVF
Dose	0.3–1 mg sublingually, tablets or spray
Contraindications/ caution	Hypersensitivity to nitrates, hypotension, hypertrophic obstructive cardiomyopathy (HOCM), aortic stenosis, cerebral trauma or stroke

Haloperidol

Indication	Agitation
Dose	2–30 mg IM
Contraindications/ caution	Coma caused by CNS depressants Dystonic reactions

Hydrocortisone

Indication	Severe asthma, anaphylaxis
Dose	200 mg IV
Contraindications/ caution	Systemic infection if no antibiotics given

Ipratropium bromide

Indication	Reversible bronchospasm in chronic obstructive pulmonary disease Reversible bronchospasm in severe bronchiolitis
Dose	250–500 μg *CHILD 125–250 μg*
Contraindications/ caution	Glaucoma

Lignocaine

Indication	Ventricular tachycardia, local anaesthesia
Dose	1 mg/kg (reduce in elderly) IV for VT
Contraindications/ caution	Hypersensitivity, epilepsy, liver disease, bradyarrhythmias, hypovolaemia Maximum dose for local anaesthesia is 3 mg/kg

Metoclopramide

Indication	Prevention of vomiting
Dose	10 mg
Contraindications/ caution	Hepatic impairment, gastrointestinal surgery Risk of dystonic reactions

Morphine

Indication	Analgesia
Dose	5–10 mg IV in 2 mg increments
	CHILD 0.1–0.2 mg/kg IV
Contraindications/ caution	Use with care in head injury or patient with decreased conscious level Have naloxone available

Nalbuphine

Indication	Analgesia
Dose	10–20 mg IV slowly in 5 mg increments *CHILD up to 300 µg/kg*
Contraindications/ caution	As with morphine May be only partially reversed by naloxone

Naloxone

Indication	Respiratory suppression due to opiates
Dose	400–12 000 µg *CHILD up to 10 µg/kg*
Contraindications/ caution	May induce acute withdrawal reaction If for overdose, give IM in case patient leaves scene

Indication	Analgesia in compliant patient who is able to self administer by inhalation. Useful in cases of isolated limb fracture or dislocation
Presentation	Blue cylinder with blue and white collar
Dose	Inhaled via a mouth piece or face mask activated by patient inspiration. The patient should be advised to take slow deep breaths. It will take 3–4 minutes to have full effect. With self administration, overdosage is prevented as deep inspiration and holding the mask cannot be maintained
Contraindications/caution	Any person needing greater than 50% oxygen, e.g. multiple trauma patient Because nitrous oxide diffuses rapidly into air filled cavities it is contra-indicated in: • possibility of pneumothorax • after recent gastro-intestinal surgery • head injury other than transient concussion (is also a cerebral vasodilator) • decompression disease
Storage	Should be kept above 6°C. Should always be shaken before use to ensure mixing of component gases.

Paracetamol

Indication	Pyrexia
Dose	*INFANT under 3 months 10 mg/kg* *3 months–1 year 60–120 mg* *1–5 years 120–250 mg* 6–12 years 250–500 mg Can be given orally or rectally
Contraindications/ caution	Liver disease

Paraldehyde

Indication	Fits not ceasing with diazemuls
Dose	Deep IM 5–10 ml or rectally in olive oil *CHILD 0.4 mg/kg rectally in* *olive oil* *Or deep IM 1–2 years 2 ml,* *3–5 years 3–4 ml, 6–12 years* *5–6 ml*
Contraindications/ caution	Hepatic impairment Sterile abscess at injection site

Prednisolone

Indication	Severe asthma
Dose	40 mg p.o.
Contraindications/ caution	Affective disorders, peptic ulcer, steroid myopathy

Salbutamol injection

Indication	Severe asthma
Dose	250–500 µg IV slowly
Contraindications/ caution	Cardiac disease, hypertension

Salbutamol nebuliser solution

Indication	Severe/moderate asthma
Dose	5 mg repeated as required
Contraindications/ caution	Cardiac disease, hypertension

Syntometrine

Indication	Post-partum haemorrhage
Dose	1 ml IM
Contraindications/ caution	Cardiac disease, multiple pregnancy

Telephone numbers

MOBILE PHONES

 Do NOT rely on your mobile phone.

- Variable coverage.
- Must switch off in A&E and critical care areas because of risk of interference with equipment.
- May be inactivated in a Major Incident (Access Control Overload: ACCOLC).
- Conversations are not recorded for future reference, unless phoning control room.

USEFUL NUMBERS/CONTACTS

Ambulance service

Duty Officer ....

Control Room Emergency Number ....

Control Room Urgent ....

HQ ....

Other ambulance service ....
Emerg Tel No ....
HQ ....
Callsign ....

Other ambulance service ....
Emerg Tel No ....
HQ ....
Callsign ....

Other ambulance service ....
Emerg Tel No ....
HQ ....
Callsign ....

Other ambulance service ....
Emerg Tel No ....
HQ ....
Callsign ....

Other ambulance service _____

Emerg Tel No _____

HQ _____

Callsign _____

Other ambulance service _____

Emerg Tel No _____

HQ _____

Callsign _____

Other ambulance service _____

Emerg Tel No _____

HQ _____

Callsign _____

Other ambulance service _____

Emerg Tel No _____

HQ _____

Callsign _____

Other ambulance service _____

Emerg Tel No _____

HQ _____

Callsign _____

Fire Control

Police Control

HM Coastguard

Mountain Rescue

RNLI

Other rescue

Hospital 1

Accident and Emergency Department

Reception ....

Fax ....

A&E Consultant ....

ext ....

Direct dial ....

A&E Emergency Line ....

ext ....

Direct dial ....

A&E Nursing station ....

ext ....

Direct dial ....

A&E Triage ....

ext ....

Direct dial ....

A&E Resus Room ....

ext ....

Direct dial ....

Major Incident Control Room ....

ext ....

Direct dial ....

Fax ....

Neurosurgical Unit ....

Hosp Tel ....

Fax ....

Burns Unit ....

Hosp Tel ....

Fax ....

Cardiothoracic Unit ....

Hosp Tel ....

Fax ....

Psychiatric Unit ....

Hosp Tel ....

Fax ....

Hospital 2

Accident and Emergency Department

Reception

Fax

A&E Consultant

ext

Direct dial

A&E Emergency Line

ext

Direct dial

A&E Nursing station

ext

Direct dial

A&E Triage

ext

Direct dial

A&E Resus Room

ext

Direct dial

Major Incident Control Room _____

ext _____

Direct dial _____

Fax _____

Neurosurgical Unit _____

Hosp Tel _____

Fax _____

Burns Unit _____

Hosp Tel _____

Fax _____

Cardiothoracic Unit _____

Hosp Tel _____

Fax _____

Psychiatric Unit _____

Hosp Tel _____

Fax _____

Hospital _____

Switchboard _____

A&E _____

Hospital _____

Switchboard _____

A&E _____

Hospital _____

Switchboard _____

A&E _____

Hospital _____

Switchboard _____

A&E _____

Hospital _____

Switchboard _____

A&E _____

Hospital _____

Switchboard _____

A&E _____

Other useful numbers

Index

Index

186